Handbook of
Oral Anticoagulation

Second edition

Handbook of Oral Anticoagulation

Second edition

Editors
Gregory YH Lip
University of Birmingham
Birmingham, UK

Eduard Shantsila
University of Birmingham
Birmingham, UK

Contributors
Deirdre A Lane
University of Birmingham
Birmingham, UK

Chee W Khoo
Specialist Registrar in Cardiology
West Midlands Deanery, UK

Kok Hoon Tay
Specialist Registrar in Cardiology
West Midlands Deanery, UK

Suresh Krishnamoorthy
Specialist Registrar in Cardiology
East Midlands Deanery, UK

Stavros Apostolakis
University of Birmingham
Birmingham, UK

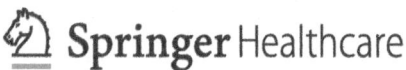

Springer Healthcare

Published by Springer Healthcare Ltd, 236 Gray's Inn Road, London, WC1X 8HB, UK.

www.springerhealthcare.com

© 2013 Springer Healthcare, a part of Springer Science+Business Media.

First edition, 2010

British Library Cataloguing-in-Publication Data.

A catalogue record for this book is available from the British Library.

ISBN 978 1 908517 58 6
eISBN 978 1 908517 96 8

Although every effort has been made to ensure that drug doses and other information are presented accurately in this publication, the ultimate responsibility rests with the prescribing physician. Neither the publisher nor the authors can be held responsible for errors or for any consequences arising from the use of the information contained herein. Any product mentioned in this publication should be used in accordance with the prescribing information prepared by the manufacturers. No claims or endorsements are made for any drug or compound at present under clinical investigation.

Project editor: Tamsin Curtis
Designer: Joe Harvey
Artworker: Sissan Mollerfors
Production: Marina Maher
Printed in Great Britain by Latimer Trend

Contents

Eduard Shantsila, Gregory YH Lip

Author biographies

Editors

Professor Gregory YH Lip is Professor of Cardiovascular Medicine at the University of Birmingham, and Visiting Professor of Haemostasis, Thrombosis, and Vascular Sciences in the School of Life and Health Sciences at the University of Aston in Birmingham, UK.

Professor Lip is a member of the scientific documents committee of the European Heart Rhythm Association (EHRA), and serves on the board of the Working Group on Hypertension of the Heart of the European Society of Cardiology (ESC). He is also a member of the Working Groups of Thrombosis and Cardiovascular Pharmacology of the ESC.

Professor Lip has acted as Clinical Adviser for the UK National Institute for Health and Clinical Excellence (NICE) guidelines on atrial fibrillation (AF) management. He was on the writing committee for the 8th American College of Chest Physicians (ACCP) Antithrombotic Therapy Guidelines for Atrial Fibrillation, as well as various guidelines and/or position statements from the EHRA, including the EHRA statement on defining endpoints for AF management, and the EHRA guidelines for antithrombotic therapy during ablation. He was also on the writing committee for the 2010 ESC Guidelines on Atrial Fibrillation and was Deputy Editor for the 9th ACCP guidelines on antithrombotic therapy for AF.

Professor Lip is involved at senior editorial level for several major international journals, including *Journal of Human Hypertension* (Editor-in-Chief), *Thrombosis and Haemostasis* (Editor-in-Chief [Clinical Studies] designate), *Thrombosis Research* (Associate Editor), *Europace* (Associate Editor), and *Circulation* (Guest Editor). He has published and lectured extensively on thrombosis and antithrombotic disease in cardiovascular disease.

Dr Eduard Shantsila is a Postdoctorate Research Fellow at the University of Birmingham Centre for Cardiovascular Science, City Hospital, Birmingham, UK, where he leads a research group working on a number of research projects that investigate endothelial damage/recovery and monocyte characteristics including their role in thrombosis in patients with acute coronary syndromes, heart failure, and systemic atherosclerosis.

Dr Shantsila worked in the Republican Research and Practical Centre 'Cardiology,' Minsk, Belarus, as a researcher and a cardiologist from 1998 and completed his PhD thesis in 2002 in Minsk, Belarus and another PhD thesis in 2012 in Birmingham, United Kingdom. From 2005 to 2008 he was a head of the Department of Urgent Cardiology in this centre, where he was actively involved in research work on the problems of cardiovascular diagnostics, endothelial dysfunction, and thrombosis. He is a member of the Working Group of Thrombosis of the ESC. Dr Shantsila has published extensively on these topics, and is a peer reviewer of major journals in thrombosis.

Contributors

Dr Stavros Apostolakis is an Honorary Lecturer in the School of Clinical and Experimental Medicine, University of Birmingham. He graduated from Medical School, University of Crete in 1999. He completed his PhD research in the same institution in 2007. He practiced medicine in Greece until October 2011. He was elected Senior Lecturer in Medicine at the Democritus University of Thrace, Greece in 2010. In the same year he was awarded the European Association of Cardiology Atherothrombosis Research Grant. His main research interests are genetic epidemiology, inflammation and coronary artery disease and atrial fibrillation.

Dr Deirdre A Lane is a Lecturer in Cardiovascular Health in the School of Clinical and Experimental Medicine at the University of Birmingham, UK. She received her Bachelor of Science with honors from the University of Liverpool in 1995 and her PhD from the University of Birmingham in 2000.

Dr Lane is currently the principal investigator on a randomized controlled trial (TREAT-ISCRTN93952605) comparing intensive education with usual care in AF patients newly referred for oral anticoagulation, to examine the impact of education on patients' knowledge and perceptions of AF and its treatment, and international normalized ratio (INR) control. In addition, she is involved in refining the risk stratification of AF patients; she is a co-author of both the CHA_2DS_2-VASc stroke risk stratification schema and HAS-BLED bleeding risk schema. She is also a panelist on the 9th edition of the American College of Chest Physicians guidelines on Antithrombotic Therapy and Prevention of Thrombosis and a member of the European Heart Rhythm Association Task Force on bleeding risk assessment in atrial fibrillation.

Dr Lane has published her work widely in journals such as *Stroke, Chest, Thrombosis and Haemostasis, Psychosomatic Medicine, Journal of Psychosomatic Research,* and *Heart.*

Dr Chee W Khoo is a Specialist Registrar in Cardiology and the West Midlands Deanery, UK. He graduated from University of Aberdeen. After successfully obtaining the MRCP. He worked at the University of Birmingham as Teaching Fellow and Cardiology Research Fellow from 2007 to 2011. His research interests are atrial fibrillation in pacemaker populations and thrombogenesis. He has published numerous articles in peer reviewed journals and also presented in national and international conferences, which include the British Cardiac Society annual conference, American College of Cardiology Conference, Heart Rhythm Congress, and the Asia–Pacific Cardio Rhythm Congress.

Dr Kok Hoon Tay is a Specialist Registrar in Cardiology and the West Midlands Deanery, UK and **Dr Suresh Krishnamoorthy** is a Specialist Registrar in Cardiology and the East Midlands Deanery, UK. They are both interested in the epidemiology and pathophysiology of thromboembolism – and the use of antithrombotic therapy – in cardiovascular disease.

Chapter 1

The coagulation pathway and approaches to anticoagulation

Kok Hoon Tay, Eduard Shantsila, Gregory YH Lip

A brief overview of the coagulation pathway

Intact endothelium is smooth, lacks thrombogenic proteins on its surface, and protects circulating blood from exposure to subendothelial proteins such as collagen. As a result, blood constituents flow freely without adhering to endothelial structures. However, when the endothelium is damaged and its integrity is disrupted, subendothelial structures come into contact with the constituents of blood (including coagulation factors and platelets), and this triggers an intricate process responsible for platelet attraction and deposition and, simultaneously, the coagulation cascade.

The coagulation cascade comprises two principal elements:

- the tissue factor (extrinsic) pathway; and
- the contact activation (intrinsic) pathway.

Both pathways ultimately lead to the formation of an insoluble fibrin clot. Each involves a series of reactions in which inactive enzyme precursors are transformed into their active forms, which catalyze the subsequent reactions of the cascade.

The fundamental role of the coagulation system is to facilitate hemostasis when there is hemorrhage due to blood vessel injury. Physiologically, a self-maintained balance of procoagulant and anticoagulant factors/regulators provides a negative feedback system for the prevention of excessive coagulation or hemorrhagic diathesis.

G. Y. H. Lip and E. Shantsila (eds.), *Handbook of Oral Anticoagulation*,
DOI: 10.1007/978-1-908517-96-8_1, © Springer Healthcare 2013

The coagulation cascade

The tissue factor (extrinsic) pathway

When the coagulation cascade is activated, tissue factor (TF), which is normally located in subendothelial tissue, comes into contact with circulating factor VII and forms an activated complex (TF–VIIa) in the presence of Ca^{2+} (Figure 1.1) [1]. TF–VIIa catalyses the conversion of factor X into factor Xa and, following binding of activated factor Va, initiates formation of the serum protease thrombin. Thrombin is formed from

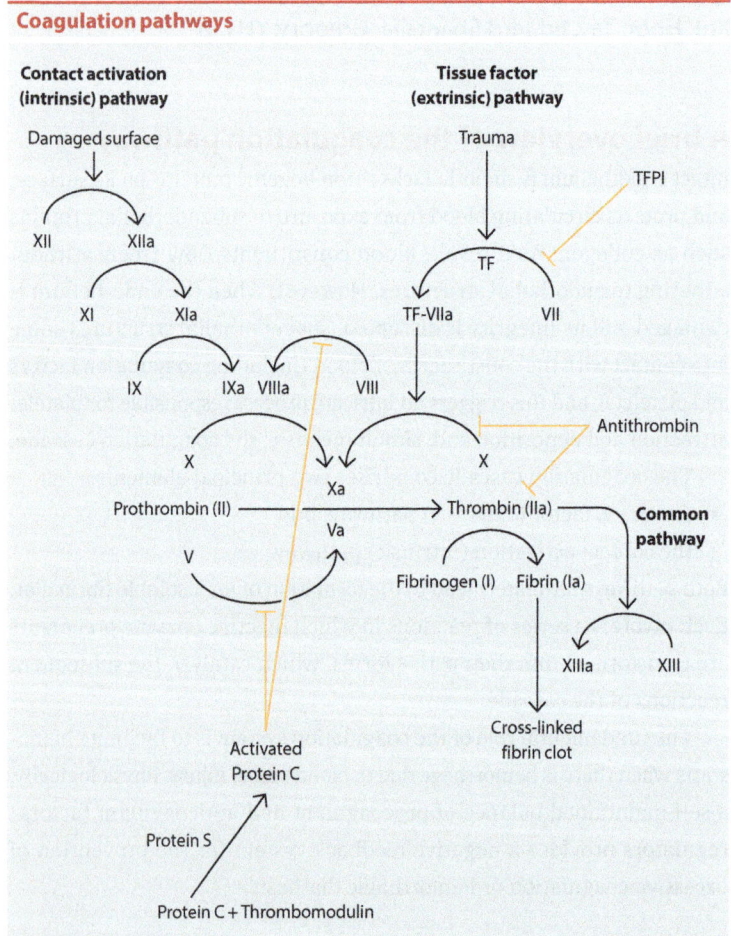

Coagulation pathways

Figure 1.1 Coagulation pathways. TFPI, Tissue factor pathway inhibitor.

prothrombin via a complex reaction in which factors Xa and Va cleave prothrombin fragments 1 and 2 in the presence of Ca^{2+}. Subsequently, thrombin cleaves fibrinopeptides A and B from fibrinogen, resulting in the formation of insoluble fibrin.

The contact activation (intrinsic) pathway

The contact activation (intrinsic) pathway begins with the formation of a complex made up of Hageman factor (factor XII), prekallikrein, high-molecular-weight kininogen (HMWK), and collagen. Given that the absence of factor XII, prekallikrein, or HMWK does not induce a clinically apparent pathology [2], the physiological role of this complex is unclear and it is assumed to have only a minor function in clot formation.

Damage to the endothelial surface triggers formation of factor XIa from factor XI via factor XIIa. Next, in the presence of Ca^{2+} factor XIa catalyses the conversion of factor IX to IXa, which then triggers the conversion of factor VIII to VIIIa. Factors IXa and VIIIa form a catalytic complex and efficiently activate factor X. Activation of factor X marks the convergence of the tissue factor and contact activation pathways into a common pathway, which is responsible for the formation of a fibrin mesh on the damaged vessel wall.

Regulation of the coagulation cascade

The 'protagonist' of the coagulation cascade is thrombin, which has a master role in regulating the coagulation pathway. Generation of thrombin subsequently activates circulating platelets bound to von Willebrand factor and factor VIIIa.

To avert excessive clotting, multiple elements of a negative feedback system maintain the coagulation cascade in a balanced state. Activated protein C (coupled with protein S) and thrombomodulin limit the excessive generation of factors Va, Xa, VIIIa, and IXa, thus both protein C and protein S act as naturally occurring anticoagulants. Antithrombin, a potent inhibitor of the coagulation cascade, inhibits thrombin and several other clotting factors involved in the cascade. Another mechanism that keeps platelet activation and coagulation under control is mediated by a TF pathway inhibitor, which has its primary role as a restrictor of TF activity.

Conclusions

The coagulation cascade is an intricate process without which hemorrhage clotting would occur uncontrollably whenever there is tissue insult.

Approaches to anticoagulation

Eduard Shantsila, Gregory YH Lip

In a large number of disorders there is a raised risk of thrombosis, the pathological development of blood clots that interfere with the circulation. Common examples include:

- venous thromboembolism, encompassing both deep vein thrombosis and pulmonary embolism;
- atrial fibrillation;
- acute coronary syndromes;
- valve disease and endocarditis; and
- conditions associated with a raised risk of ischemic stroke.

The coagulation cascade is a major target for thromboprophylactic medications. Anticoagulation can be achieved by inhibition of different factors of coagulation. For example, warfarin, discussed in Chapter 3, reduces the functional level of factors II (prothrombin), VII, IX, and X by preventing the γ-carboxylation of these vitamin K-dependent factors. However, a disadvantage of warfarin and other vitamin K antagonists is that they are associated with a raised risk of hemorrhage, as described in Chapter 4, together with the fact that their effect fluctuates in any one patient and necessitates frequent monitoring.

Another route exploited for anticoagulation is the use of heparin to increase the inhibitory action of antithrombin. Heparin preparations are the mainstay of anticoagulation in many clinical settings, as reviewed in Chapter 2. However, unlike warfarin, heparin preparations require parenteral administration.

The ideal anticoagulant would be an oral preparation that has a more predictable therapeutic action and which requires significantly less monitoring than warfarin. Consequently, the development of a number of alternative oral anticoagulants is of great interest. Modern novel anticoagulant development has focused on the synthesis of selective inhibitors of specific coagulation factors, which preferably act independently of cofactors. Novel oral anticoagulants targeting inhibition of factor Xa and thrombin (factor IIa) have now been incorporated into clinical practice, as discussed in Chapter 5. These factors are the final elements of the coagulation cascade and their inhibition blocks both the intrinsic (plasma) and the extrinsic (tissue) coagulation cascades.

References

1   Mann KG, Nesheim ME, Church WR, et al. Surface-dependent reactions of the vitamin K dependent enzyme complexes. *Blood*. 1990;76:1-16.

2   Badimon L, Badimon JJ. The pathophysiology of thrombus. In: Blann A, Lip GYH, Turpie AGG (eds), *Thrombosis in Clinical Practice*. London: Taylor & Francis; 2005:1-16.

Chapter 2

Common clinical indications for anticoagulation

Suresh Krishnamoorthy, Chee W Khoo, Eduard Shantsila, Gregory YH Lip

As discussed in Chapter 1, an anticoagulant is a substance that possesses the properties to limit clot formation and therefore can be used therapeutically to prevent or treat thrombotic disorders. In this chapter we discuss the common clinical conditions in which anticoagulation should be considered and the evidence available to justify the use of an appropriate antithrombotic therapy in these clinical settings.

Venous thromboembolism

Epidemiology

Venous thromboembolism (VTE) encompasses both deep vein thrombosis (DVT) and pulmonary embolism (PE). It is a common disorder with an incidence of 7.1 per 1000 person-years in developed countries [1,2]. VTE is more common in males and in black populations, and the incidence increases with aging. Furthermore, up to a fifth of patients with previous VTE have recurrences of VTE in the following 5 years [3].

PE, a life-threatening presentation of VTE, has a reported incidence of 6 cases per 10,000 person-years [4]. Notably, around 80% of cases of PE occur without any clinical signs [5]. It is also estimated that 1 in every 100 inpatient deaths is related to PE, making it one of the most common causes of preventable hospital mortality [6].

G. Y. H. Lip and E. Shantsila (eds.), *Handbook of Oral Anticoagulation*,
DOI: 10.1007/978-1-908517-96-8_2, © Springer Healthcare 2013

Given that patients with VTE have a substantially increased risk of morbidity and mortality because of its complications (life-threatening PE and post-thrombotic syndrome) [7], when its presence is suspected patients should be carefully considered to ensure timely diagnosis and initiation of treatment. Common conditions associated with VTE are shown in Table 2.1. The imbalance between the activated coagulation cascade (both intrinsic and extrinsic pathways) and the fibrinolytic system is another predisposing feature that increases the risk of VTE.

It is worth mentioning that venous thrombi differ in site of formation and are rich in red cells compared with arterial thrombi, which are mainly platelet rich. Consequently, the antithrombotic effects of anticoagulants may vary substantially depending on thrombus location and these agents require a specific regimen for the clinical settings of venous thrombosis (eg, VTE) and arterial thrombosis (eg, acute coronary syndromes).

Anticoagulation in the prevention of venous thromboembolism

The incidence of VTE can be reduced significantly using prophylactic regimens in high-risk patients. Appropriate prophylaxis has been found to be cost-effective compared with the cost of managing established VTE cases [8].

Various prophylactic measures have been recommended in the prevention of VTE, including injections of low-dose unfractionated heparin (UFH), adjusted-dose UFH, low-molecular-weight heparin (LMWH), oral warfarin, external pneumatic compression, or gradient elastic stockings

Common conditions associated with venous thromboembolism

Post-trauma

- Post-surgical patients (major surgery lasting >30 min, orthopedic surgeries)
- Previous deep vein thrombosis/pulmonary embolism
- Prolonged immobilization (bed rest, paralysis of legs or plaster casts, long flights)
- Malignancy
- Obesity
- Pregnancy, use of oral contraceptive pills
- Advanced age
- Other conditions: antithrombin III deficiency, protein C and S deficiency (eg, varicose veins, thrombocytosis, polycythemia rubra vera, systemic lupus erythematosus, nephritic syndrome, stroke and debilitating infections)

Table 2.1 Common conditions associated with venous thromboembolism.

alone or in combination. Prophylactic therapy in high-risk patients should be tailored carefully, assessing both individual risk(s) and therapeutic benefits. Nevertheless, in contrast to the management of developed thrombosis, prophylactic therapy is simple, carries minimal risks and, if warfarin is not used, does not require monitoring.

In a meta-analysis of trials (n=19,958) using parenteral anticoagulant thromboprophylaxis (UFH, LMWH, fondaparinux) in hospitalized medical patients, there was a significant risk reduction in PE (relative risk [RR] 0.43, 95% confidence interval [CI] 0.26–0.71) and fatal PE (RR 0.38, 95% CI 0.21–0.69) and a nonsignificant reduction in DVT (RR 0.47, 95% CI 0.22–1.00) [9]. There was no effect on all-cause mortality (RR 0.97, 95% CI 0.790–1.19), and, impressively, there was no significant increase in the risk of major hemorrhage (RR 1.32, 95% CI 0.73–2.37).

From another meta-analysis of randomized trials (n=16,000), perioperative use of prophylactic low-dose UFH reduced the incidence of DVT (odds ratio [OR] 0.3), symptomatic PE (OR 0.5), fatal PE (OR 0.4), and all-cause mortality (OR 0.8) compared with placebo in those undergoing general, orthopedic, and urological surgery [10]. In another analysis, there was an increase in the incidence of wound hematomas with low-dose UFH compared with placebo, although the incidence of major hemorrhage in these patients was not increased [11]. However, the use of UFH is limited due to its shorter half-life and the requirement for repeated injections and monitoring of the activated partial thromboplastin time (APTT).

Because of these limitations, there has been a major switch in clinical practice from low-dose UFH to LMWH (depolymerized UFH). This has both clinical and practical advantages: LMWH has a longer half-life, has higher bioavailability, and can be safely administered subcutaneously without the need for monitoring. In one meta-analysis, LMWH prophylaxis in patients undergoing general surgery showed a reduction of up to 70% in asymptomatic DVT and symptomatic VTE compared with no prophylaxis [12]. In a meta-analysis assessing the efficacy of individual anticoagulant agents, LMWH appeared to be more effective than UFH in the prevention of asymptomatic DVT (RR 0.47, 95% CI 0.36–0.62), without any increased risk of thrombocytopenia or hemorrhage [13], and it was also more cost-effective than UFH [14]. Similarly, meta-analyses of head-to-head trials comparing LMWH and UFH prophylaxis in patients undergoing abdominal, hip, or knee surgery showed superior efficacy for LMWH in reducing VTE and deaths related to VTE with a good safety profile [15–17].

Hopes for a further improvement in parenteral management of thrombosis were associated with the introduction of the selective indirect factor Xa inhibitor fondaparinux. However, although the benefits of fondaparinux were demonstrated in patients with acute coronary syndromes, it has been found to have similar effectiveness and safety to the LMWH dalteparin in patients undergoing high-risk abdominal surgery [18].

Oral anticoagulants for thromboprophylaxis after surgery

Until recently, oral anticoagulants were not considered an option for thromboprophylaxis after surgery. Warfarin could not be recommended for VTE prevention due to its delayed onset of action, its narrow therapeutic range and the requirement for careful monitoring. The novel oral direct thrombin inhibitor ximelagatran achieved favorable results in initial trials but was removed from further development because of safety issues [19,20]. More recently, however, newer oral anticoagulants have been shown to be safe and effective for thromboprophylaxis after surgery (see Chapter 5).

Guidelines for prevention of venous thromboembolism

The risk of VTE is not homogeneous and depends on the presence of concomitant risk factors. The American College of Chest Physicians (ACCP) has published evidence-based clinical practice guidelines on VTE prevention following surgery and other medical conditions (Tables 2.2–2.4) [21].

Treatment of venous thromboembolism

A number of randomized trials have confirmed that in patients with lower-limb DVT, LMWH is superior to UFH in reducing mortality at 3–6 months and reducing the risk of hemorrhage [22]. Furthermore, a meta-analysis of trials comparing UFH and LMWH for the treatment of VTE showed no difference in the recurrence of VTE or PE, in minor or major hemorrhage, or in thrombocytopenia [23]. Furthermore, a 24% reduction in the risk of total mortality was observed in patients treated with LMWH compared with UFH (RR 0.76, 95% CI 0.59–0.98). Treatment of PE with LMWH also appears to be safe, being at least as effective as UFH, and also cost effective, without the need for special laboratory monitoring [24,25]. LMWHs have also proved to be effective and safe options for the outpatient treatment of VTE [26–28].

Prevention of venous thromboembolism in non-surgical patients

Condition	Recommendations
Acutely ill hospitalized medical patients at increased risk of thrombosis	LMWH, LDUH, or fondaparinux (Grade 1B)
For acutely ill hospitalized medical patients at low risk of thrombosis, or who are bleeding or at high risk for bleeding	No prophylaxis (Grade 1B)
Acutely ill hospitalized medical patients at increased risk of thrombosis who are bleeding or at high risk for major bleeding	Mechanical thromboprophylaxis with GCS or IPC (Grade 2C)
Critically ill patients with no bleeding	LMWH or LDUH thromboprophylaxis (Grade 2C)
Critically ill patients, who are bleeding, or are at high risk for major bleeding	Mechanical thromboprophylaxis with GCS or IPC (Grade 2C)
Outpatients with cancer who have no additional risk factors for VTE*	No routine prophylaxis (Grade 1B)
Outpatients with solid tumors who have additional risk factors for VTE and who are at low risk of bleeding*	Prophylactic dose LMWH or LDUH (Grade 2B)
Outpatients with cancer and indwelling central venous catheters	No routine prophylaxis (Grade 2B for LMWH or LDUH, Grade 2C for VKAs)
Chronically immobilized persons residing at home or at a nursing home	No routine prophylaxis (Grade 2C)
Long-distance travelers at increased risk of VTE†	Frequent ambulation, calf muscle exercise, or sitting in an aisle seat if feasible; below knee GCS (Grade 2C)
Asymptomatic thrombophilia	No long-term daily use mechanical or pharmacologic thromboprophylaxis to prevent VTE (Grade 1C)

Table 2.2 Prevention of venous thromboembolism in non-surgical patients. These recommendations are from the American College of Chest Physicians evidence-based clinical practice guidelines. *Additional risk factors for venous thrombosis in cancer outpatients include previous venous thrombosis, immobilization, hormonal therapy, angiogenesis inhibitors, thalidomide, and lenalidomide. †Increased risk of VTE includes previous VTE, recent surgery or trauma, active malignancy, pregnancy, estrogen use, advanced age, limited mobility, severe obesity, or known thrombophilic disorder). GCS, gradient compression stockings; IPC, intermittent pneumatic compression; LDUH, low-dose unfractionated heparin; LMWH, low-molecular-weight heparin; VKA, vitamin K antagonist; VTE, venous thromboembolism. Data from Guyatt et al [21].

Prevention of venous thromboembolism in non-orthopedic surgical patients

Conditions	Recommendations
General and abdominal-pelvic surgery	
Very low risk for VTE*	No pharmacologic (Grade 1B) or mechanical (Grade 2C) prophylaxis
Low risk for VTE	Mechanical prophylaxis (Grade 2C)
Moderate risk for VTE (not at high risk for major bleeding)	LMWH (Grade 2B), LDUH (Grade 2B), or mechanical prophylaxis (Grade 2C)
Moderate risk for VTE (at high risk for major bleeding or with bleeding thought to have particularly severe consequences)	Mechanical prophylaxis (Grade 2C)
High risk for VTE (not at high risk for major bleeding)	LMWH (Grade 1B) or LDUH (Grade 1B). Plus mechanical prophylaxis (Grade 2C)
High-VTE-risk patients undergoing surgery for cancer (not at high risk for major bleeding)	Extended (4 weeks) LMWH (Grade 1B)
High-VTE-risk patients (at high risk for major bleeding or with bleeding thought to have particularly severe consequences)	Mechanical prophylaxis (Grade 2C)
High risk for VTE in whom both LMWH and UFH are contraindicated or unavailable (not at high risk for major bleeding)	Low-dose aspirin, fondaparinux, or mechanical prophylaxis (Grade 2C)
Cardiac surgery	
Uncomplicated	Mechanical prophylaxis (Grade 2C)
Hospital course is prolonged nonhemorrhagic surgical complications	Pharmacologic prophylaxis (LDUH or LMWH) and mechanical prophylaxis (Grade 2C)
Thoracic surgery	
Moderate risk for VTE (not at high risk for perioperative bleeding)	LDUH or LMWH (Grade 2B), or mechanical prophylaxis with IPC (Grade 2C)
High risk for VTE (not at high risk for perioperative bleeding)	LDUH or LMWH (Grade 1B). Plus mechanical prophylaxis (Grade 2C)
High risk for major bleeding	Mechanical prophylaxis (Grade 2C)
Craniotomy	
At very high risk for VTE (eg, those undergoing craniotomy for malignant disease)	Pharmacologic prophylaxis added once adequate hemostasis is established and the risk of bleeding decreases (Grade 2C)
Spinal surgery at high risk for VTE (including those with malignant disease or those undergoing surgery with a combined anterior-posterior approach)	Mechanical prophylaxis (Grade 2C), UFH (Grade 2C), or LMWH (Grade 2C)

Table 2.3 Prevention of venous thromboembolism in non-orthopedic surgical patients (continues opposite).

Prevention of venous thromboembolism in non-orthopedic surgical patients (continued)

Major trauma

Low risk for VTE	LDUH, LMWH, or mechanical prophylaxis (Grade 2C)
High risk for VTE (including those with acute spinal cord injury, traumatic brain injury, and spinal surgery for trauma)	Adding mechanical prophylaxis to pharmacologic prophylaxis (Grade 2C) when not contraindicated by leg injury
If LMWH and LDUH are contraindicated	Mechanical prophylaxis (Grade 2C) when not contraindicated by leg injury

Table 2.3 Prevention of venous thromboembolism in non-orthopedic surgical patients (continued). These recommendations are from the American College of Chest Physicians evidence-based clinical practice guidelines. *Based on Rogers and Caprini scores. LDUH, low-dose unfractionated heparin; LMWH, low-molecular-weight heparin; UFH, unfractionated heparin; VTE, venous thromboembolism. Data from Guyatt et al [21].

Prevention of venous thromboembolism in patients undergoing major orthopedic surgery

Total hip arthroplasty or total knee arthroplasty
One of the following for a minimum of 10 to 14 days: LMWH, fondaparinux, apixaban, dabigatran, rivaroxaban, LDUH, VKA, aspirin (Grade 1B), or IPCD (Grade 1C)

LMWH is preferred to other agents for THA and TKA: fondaparinux, apixaban, dabigatran, rivaroxaban, LDUH (all Grade 2B), adjusted-dose VKA, or aspirin (all Grade 2C)

Hip fracture surgery
One of the following for a minimum of 10 to 14 days: LMWH, fondaparinux, LDUH, VKA, aspirin (Grade 1B), or an IPCD (Grade 1C)

LMWH is preferred to the other agents (fondaparinux, LDUH [Grade 2B]; adjusted-dose VKA or aspirin [Grade 2C])

Major orthopedic surgery: total hip arthroplasty, total knee arthroplasty and hip fracture surgery
If receiving LMWH as thromboprophylaxis, to start either ≥12 hours preoperatively or ≥12 hours postoperatively rather than within ≤4 hours preoperatively or ≤4 hours postoperatively (Grade 1B)

Extend thromboprophylaxis in the outpatient period for up to 35 days from the day of surgery (Grade 2B)

Use dual prophylaxis with an antithrombotic agent and an IPCD during the hospital stay (Grade 2C)

If increased risk of bleeding, use an IPCD or no prophylaxis rather than pharmacologic treatment (Grade 2C)

If patients declines or is uncooperative with injections or an IPCD, use apixaban or dabigatran (if both are unavailable then rivaroxaban or VKA), all (Grade 1B)

Table 2.4 Prevention of venous thromboembolism in patients undergoing major orthopedic surgery. These recommendations are from the American College of Chest Physicians evidence-based clinical practice guidelines. IPCD, intermittent pneumatic compression device; LDUH, low-dose unfractionated heparin; LMWH, low-molecular-weight heparin; VKA, vitamin K antagonist. Data from Guyatt et al [21].

In the MATISSE-DVT (Mondial Assessment of Thromboembolism treatment Initiated by Synthetic pentasaccharide with Symptomatic Endpoints – Deep Vein Thrombosis) trial [29], once-daily subcutaneous administration of fondaparinux was found to be noninferior to twice-daily injection of the LMWH enoxaparin, with no differences in the recurrence of DVT, major hemorrhage or death at 3 months.

A disadvantage of LMWHs is that they require daily subcutaneous injections, often by trained personnel. Consequently, oral anticoagulation is considered an attractive option. Available data indicate that warfarin is non-inferior to LMWH in patients with VTE (without cancers), with a similar rate of VTE recurrence or hemorrhage [30]. Of interest, these positive results with warfarin were noted despite patients spending a relatively low proportion of time within the therapeutic international normalized ratio (INR) range, thus mirroring real life primary care practice. However, in patients with coexistent malignancies, treatment with LMWH appears to be more efficacious compared with warfarin [31].

Decisions with regard to the duration of warfarin anticoagulation in patients with VTE should be guided by whether or not the etiology is idiopathic. In many trials the VTE patient cohorts have been highly heterogeneous; nevertheless, it is clear from the pooled analyses that, compared with early termination of treatment, prolonged anticoagulation with warfarin (INR 2–3) is associated with a significant reduction in the recurrence of VTE [32–34], albeit with a nonsignificant increase in the risk of hemorrhage. Conventional intensity warfarin therapy (INR 2–3) has also been found to be more effective than low-intensity (INR 1.5–2) warfarin anticoagulation [35,36], without any increased risk of hemorrhage in patients with symptomatic VTE.

The indirect factor Xa inhibitor idraparinux (injected subcutaneously once weekly) was found in a randomized trial [37] to be as effective and safe as warfarin in patients with VTE, with no differences in DVT recurrence. However, idraparinux was comparatively less effective in patients with PE, and long-term therapy carried higher hemorrhage risks than did warfarin.

As an alternative to oral and parenteral anticoagulation for VTE management, catheter-directed thrombolysis [38–40] and thrombus removal [41] can be used and have been shown to improve the venous patency and outcomes in patients with acute DVT. By contrast, the available evidence for the utility of inferior vena cava filters [42,43] for treatment of VTE is conflicting, and therefore their routine use is not recommended. If they are used, patients should also receive conventional anticoagulation treatment. With regard to thrombolysis in acute PE, a meta-analysis of trials comparing thrombolysis with heparin showed a nonsignificant reduction in PE recurrence (OR 0.67, 95% CI 0.4–1.12) and all-cause mortality (OR 0.70, 95% CI 0.37–1.30) with thrombolysis, but this was achieved at the expense of a significant increase in nonmajor hemorrhage (OR 2.63, 95% CI 1.53–4.54) and intracranial hemorrhages [44].

Guidelines for treatment of venous thromboembolism

Current guidelines recommend long-term oral anticoagulation at a conventional intensity (INR 2–3 for vitamin K antagonist [VKA]) for patients with VTE (Table 2.5) [21,45]. The duration of the treatment should be 3–6 months in those with precipitating risk factors and 12 months for 'idiopathic' VTE; however, in the event of further recurrences, the therapy should be further extended (for 12 months or more). Thrombolysis in patients with PE is reserved for those with hemodynamic instability or with other poor prognostic features, such as hypoxia, dilated and hypokinetic right ventricle, or elevated cardiac markers. Importantly, precipitating factors, such as occult malignancies (4–10% of VTE cases) [46], should be carefully considered in VTE patients, particularly in those with 'idiopathic' VTE.

In patients with acute VTE warfarin should be immediately initiated together with parenteral anticoagulation. Parenteral anticoagulation (LMWH of fondaparinux) should be used for at least 5 days and should not be discontinued until the INR reaches 2.0 for at least 24 hours. First episodes of VTE should be managed with an INR target of 2.5 (2.0–2.5), while more advanced anticoagulation should be employed with a target of INR 3.5 (3.0–4.0) in patients with recurrent VTE [21].

Current guidelines for the treatment of venous thromboembolism

Condition	Anticoagulation
Acute DVT	
Initial treatment	Parenteral anticoagulants (LMWH, fondaparinux, or UFH) (Grade 1B)
Long-term treatment	Adjusted VKA (INR 2–3) (Grade 1B)
DVT provoked by surgery or by a nonsurgical transient risk factor	3 months (Grade 1B)
First unprovoked proximal DVT (low or moderate bleeding risk)	Extended (Grade 2B)*
First unprovoked proximal DVT (high bleeding risk)	3 months (Grade 1B)†
First unprovoked isolated distal DVT	3 months (Grade 2B if a low or moderate bleeding, Grade 1B a high bleeding risk)†
Second unprovoked VTE (low or moderate bleeding risk)	Extended (Grade 1B if low bleeding risk, Grade 2B if a moderate bleeding risk)*
Second unprovoked VTE (high bleeding risk)	3 months (Grade 2B)†
Any DVT and active cancer	Extended (Grade 1B if non high bleeding risk, Grade 2B if a high bleeding risk)*
Acute PE	
Initial treatment	Parenteral anticoagulants and VKA (Grade 1B). Parenteral anticoagulation for a minimum of 5 days and until the INR is 2.0 or above for at least 24 hours (Grade 1B)
If hypotension or high risk of hypotension and no high bleeding risk	Systemic thrombolysis (Grade 2C)
Long-term treatment	Adjusted VKA (INR 2–3) (Grade 1B)
PE provoked by surgery or by a nonsurgical transient risk factor	3 months (Grade 1B)
First unprovoked PE (low or moderate bleeding risk)	Extended (Grade 2B)*
First unprovoked PE of the leg (high bleeding risk)	3 months (Grade 1B)†
Second unprovoked VTE (low or moderate bleeding risk)	Extended (Grade 1B if low bleeding risk, Grade 2B if a moderate bleeding risk)*
Second unprovoked VTE (high bleeding risk)	3 months (Grade 2B)†
Any PE and active cancer	Extended (Grade 1B if low or moderate bleeding risk, Grade 2B if high bleeding risk)*

Table 2.5 Current guidelines for the treatment of venous thromboembolism. DVT, deep vein thrombosis; INR, international normalized ratio; LMWH, low-molecular-weight heparin; PE, pulmonary embolism; VKA, vitamin K antagonist; UFH, unfractionated heparin. *The continuing use of treatment should be reassessed at periodic intervals (eg, annually). †The risk–benefit ratio of extended therapy should be reassessed after 3 months. Data from Guyatt et al [21] and Keeling [45].

Atrial fibrillation

Epidemiology and thromboembolic risks with atrial fibrillation

The overall prevalence of atrial fibrillation (AF) was 6% in the Framingham and Rotterdam studies [47,48]. Both of these studies found a one in four lifetime risk of developing AF, for both men and women aged 40 years and above. The population-based Renfrew–Paisley study in west Scotland found the prevalence of AF among patients aged 45–64 years to be 6.5% [49]; the prevalence of AF increases with age and is higher in males. The incidence of AF has risen by 13% over the past two decades, and it is predicted that 15.9 million people in the USA will have AF by 2050 [50].

The clinical significance of AF is largely associated with its increased risk for thromboembolic complications. The risk of ischemic stroke or thromboembolism is four- to five-fold higher across all age groups in patients with AF, and is similar in patients with either paroxysmal or permanent AF [51].

Acute atrial fibrillation

At present no clinical trial data are available that assesses the role of anticoagulation in acute AF with hemodynamic instability. Consensus statements made by the UK National Institute for Health and Clinical Excellence (NICE) and the European Society of Cardiology (ESC) guidelines (2010) [54] advocate the use of heparin prior to cardioversion in acute AF, irrespective of the method used. In a randomized clinical trial of 155 patients with AF duration between 2 and 19 days and who were undergoing transesophageal echocardiograph-guided cardioversion, no significant differences between UFH and LMWH were observed in rates of stroke, systemic embolism, thrombus formation, or hemorrhage [55]. The use of LMWH simplifies the treatment regimen and allows early discharge from hospital [56]; however, for patients with planned cardioversion (whether electrical or pharmacological), oral anticoagulation has to be initiated and therapeutic levels maintained for at least 3 weeks before and 4 weeks after the procedure.

Long-term oral anticoagulation should be considered in patients with stroke risk factors or if there is a high risk of AF recurrence. If successful cardioversion has not been achieved, the need for long-term thrombo-prophylaxis should be assessed according to the patient's individual stroke risk.

Long-term thromboprophylaxis

The long-term risk of stroke is not homogeneous among AF patients. Each patient with AF should be assessed for thromboembolic risk, contrain-dications, and comorbidities prior to commencement of antithrombotic therapy [55]. The state-of-the-art approach for anticoagulation in AF has been presented in the updated guidelines of the ESC on management of this disorder [52]. These recommendations include the introduction of a more advanced system of stroke-risk stratification.

The guidelines recommend to perform an initial rapid risk assess-ment using the simplest risk assessment scheme called the CHADS2 score (Cardiac failure, Hypertension, Age ≥75 years, Diabetes, Stroke [2 points]) based on a point system in which 2 points are assigned for a history of stroke or transitory ischemic attack and 1 point each for other risk factors. Life-long oral anticoagulation therapy should be initiated in patients with a CHADS2 score ≥2 (INR target of 2.5 [range, 2.0–3.0]), unless contraindicated.

A more detailed stroke risk-assessment schema is recommended in subjects with CHADS2 scores 0–1, which considers both 'major' and 'clinically relevant nonmajor' stroke risk factors. This new schema is abbreviated as CHA_2DS_2-VASc (Congestive heart failure, Hypertension, Age ≥75 [doubled], Diabetes, Stroke [doubled], Vascular disease, Age 65–74, and Sex category [female]) (Table 2.6) [56]. Patients with 1 'major' or >2 'clinically relevant nonmajor' risk factors are considered high-risk and should receive oral anticoagulant therapy. In patients with one 'clinically relevant nonmajor' risk factor antithrombotic therapy is recommended either as oral anticoagulant therapy (INR 2.0–3.0) or aspirin 75–325 mg daily. Patients with no risk factors, such as those aged <65 years with lone AF, should receive aspirin 75–325 mg daily or no antithrombotic therapy at all.

It is important to point out that the same approach towards antico-agulation should be applied to subjects with paroxysmal, persistent, or

Stroke and bleeding risk assessment: the CHA$_2$DS$_2$-VASc schema for stroke risk assessment

	Clinical characteristics	Clinical characteristics
C	Congestive heart failure/LV dysfunction	1
H	Hypertension	1
A$_2$	Age ≥75 years	2
D	Diabetes mellitus	1
S$_2$	Stroke/TIA/TE	2
V	Vascular disease	1
A	Age 65–74 years	1
Sc	Sex category (ie, female gender)	1
		Maximum 9 points

Table 2.6 Stroke and bleeding risk assessment: the CHA$_2$DS$_2$-VASc schema for stroke risk assessment. In patients with thyrotoxicosis, antithrombotic therapy should be chosen based on the presence of other stroke risk factors, as listed in this figure. 'Vascular disease' refers to myocardial infarction, complex aortic plaque, and PAD, including prior revascularization, amputation due to PAD or angiographic evidence of PAD. LV, left ventricular; PAD, peripheral artery disease; TE, thromboembolic event; TIA, transient ischemic attack. Data from Lip et al [56]. © 2010, American College of Chest Physicians.

permanent AF and those with atrial flutter. Subjects with AF who have mechanical heart valves should receive chronic oral anticoagulation based on the type and position of the prosthesis, with INR of at least 2.5 in the mitral position and at least 2.0 for an aortic valve.

While warfarin is still the most commonly used oral anticoagulant, novel non-VKA anticoagulants have been recently introduced and will be discussed in detail in Chapter 5. Additionally the risk of bleeding associated with chronic oral anticoagulation in AF should not be neglected. Approaches for individual assessment of risk of bleeding have been validated and introduced into clinical practice recently and are discussed in Chapter 4.

Warfarin versus placebo

The clinical trials that have compared warfarin with either control or placebo are summarized in Table 2.7 [55,57–61]. The results of these trials and a meta-analysis of adjusted-dose warfarin in AF patients showed a two-thirds reduction, compared with placebo, in the relative risk of ischemic stroke or systemic embolism in high-risk patients [62,63].

Thromboprophylaxis in atrial fibrillation: clinical trials comparing warfarin with control

Study	Number of patients (warfarin)	Target INR	Thromboembolic event/patients, warfarin vs placebo	RRR (%); comments
AFASAK [55]	671 (335)	2.8–4.2	5/335 vs 21/336	54
BAATAF [57]	420 (212)	1.5–2.7	3/212 vs 13/208	78
CAFA [58]	378 (187)	2.0–3.0	6/187 vs 9/191	33
EAFT [59] (secondary prevention study)	439 (225)	2.5–4.0	20/225 vs 50/214	68; mean follow-up 2.3 years; annual rate of outcome event was 8% vs 17%
SPAF-I [60]	421 (210)	2.0–4.5	8/210 vs 19/211	60
SPINAF [61]	571 (281)	1.4–2.8	7/281 vs 23/290	70; mean follow up 1.8 years; annual event rate among patients over 70 years of age: 4.8% in placebo group, 0.9% in warfarin group (risk reduction 0.79)

Table 2.7 Thromboprophylaxis in atrial fibrillation: clinical trials comparing warfarin with control. AFASAK, Atrial Fibrillation, Aspirin, Anticoagulation trial; BAATAF, Boston Area Anticoagulation Trial for Atrial Fibrillation; CAFA, Canadian Atrial Fibrillation Anticoagulation trial; EAFT, European Atrial Fibrillation Trial; INR, international normalized ratio; RRR, relative risk reduction; SPAF, Stroke Prevention in Atrial Fibrillation trial; SPINAF, Stroke Prevention in Non-rheumatic Atrial Fibrillation trial. Data from [55,57–61].

Aspirin versus placebo

The clinical trials that have compared antiplatelet therapy with either placebo or control are summarized in Table 2.8 [55,59,60,64–67]. Various aspirin doses between 50 and 1200 mg daily have been employed in these trials and evaluated during follow-up periods ranging from 1.2 years to 4.0 years. Recent meta-analyses have reported that antiplatelet drugs, when compared with controls, reduced overall stroke risk by 19–22% [62,68]. However, this magnitude of stroke reduction is similar to that seen with the use of antiplatelet therapy in high-risk vascular disorders and, given that AF commonly coexists with vascular disease, the effect of aspirin may simply reflect the effect on vascular disease.

Warfarin versus antiplatelet therapy

A meta-analysis of 12 large randomized trials involving 12,721 participants found a 39% RR reduction in all strokes when INR-adjusted-dose warfarin

Thromboprophylaxis in atrial fibrillation: clinical trials comparing aspirin with control

Study	Number of patients (aspirin)	Doses (mg/day)	Thromboembolic event/ patients	RRR (%); comments
AFASAK [55]	672 (336)	75	16/336 vs 19/336	17
EAFT [59]	782 (404)	300	88/404 vs 90/378	11
ESPS [64]	211 (104)	50	17/104 vs 23/107	At mean follow-up of 2 years. Stroke risk was reduced by 18% with aspirin compared with placebo
SPAF-I [60]	1120 (552)	325	25/552 vs 44/568	44
UK-TIA [65]	(a) 28 (13) (b) 36 (21)	300 1200	3/13 vs 4/15 5/21 vs 4/15	17 14
JAST [66]	871 (426)	150	20/426 vs 19/445	10
LASAF [67]	(a) 195 (104) (b) 181 (90)	125 125 mg/ alt day	4/104 vs 3/91 1/90 vs 3/91	17 67

Table 2.8 Thromboprophylaxis in atrial fibrillation: clinical trials comparing aspirin with control. AFASAK, Atrial Fibrillation, Aspirin, Anticoagulation trial; alt, alternate; EAFT, European Atrial Fibrillation Trial; ESPS, European Stroke Prevention Study; JAST, Japan Atrial Fibrillation Stroke Trial; LASAF, Low-dose Aspirin, Stroke, Atrial Fibrillation; RRR, relative risk reduction; SPAF, Stroke Prevention in Atrial Fibrillation trial; UK-TIA, United Kingdom Transient Ischaemic Attack. Data from [55,59,60,64–67].

was compared with aspirin [62]. Clopidogrel plus aspirin versus oral anticoagulation for AF in the Atrial fibrillation Clopidogrel Trial with Irbesartan for prevention of Vascular Events (ACTIVE-W) [69], the largest of these trials, was stopped early because of the clear evidence of superiority of adjusted-dose warfarin.

In the randomized Birmingham Atrial Fibrillation Treatment of the Aged (BAFTA) study [70], warfarin (INR 2–3) was compared with aspirin 75 mg daily in 973 patients with AF aged 75 years or older in a primary care setting. The study demonstrated that during the average 2.7-year follow-up warfarin was significantly more effective than aspirin in preventing stroke (by over 50%, with nearly 2% annual absolute risk reduction), without any difference between warfarin and aspirin in the risk of major hemorrhage.

At present, adjusted-dose warfarin remains the most efficacious prophylaxis for AF patients who have at least moderate risk of stroke.

Anticoagulation in other medical conditions

Valve disease and endocarditis

In patients with prosthetic mechanical heart valves, oral anticoagulation offers superior and consistent protection against systemic thromboembolism compared with antiplatelet agents and is therefore recommended in all such patients [71]. VKA are medications of choice in patients with mechanical cardiac prosthetic valves. Novel oral anticoagulants should not be used in patients with a mechanical prosthesis, due to lack of evidence of their effectiveness and safety in these settings [72].

Target INR is established based on the presence of risk factors and the thrombogenicity of the prosthesis. Carbomedics, Medtronic Hall, St Jude Medical and ON-X prostheses have low thrombogenicity; other bileaflet valves have medium thrombogenicity, whilst Lillehei-Kaster, Omniscience, Starr-Edwards, Bjork-Shiley and other tilting-disc valves pose high risk of thrombogenicity. The target median INR should be 2.5, 3.0, and 3.5 for prostheses with low, medium, and high thrombogenicity, respectively. The target INR values should be increased by 0.5 in a patient who has one or more of the following patient-related risk factors: mitral or tricuspid valve replacement; previous thromboembolism; atrial fibrillation; mitral stenosis of any degree; left ventricular ejection fraction 35%. The target INR recommendations may need to be reduced if recurrent bleeding occurs, or increased in cases of embolism that has developed despite an acceptable INR level. Low-dose aspirin rather than anticoagulants is now considered as a preferable option in patients after aortic bioprostheses [72].

Both infective and nonbacterial thrombotic endocarditis carry a higher risk of embolic stroke. Persistent vegetation of >10 mm despite treatment, or one or more embolic events in the first 2 weeks of treatment, are indications for acute surgical treatment of the affected valves [73]. Nevertheless, data on the benefits of anticoagulant drugs in these clinical settings are lacking.

Acute myocardial infarction, left ventricular thrombus, and aneurysm

The risk of stroke associated with acute myocardial infarction (MI) accompanied by left ventricular (LV) mural thrombus can be as high as

15% [74]. Nearly half of all patients with LV aneurysm have LV thrombus, and in such patients the extent of MI, severity of LV dysfunction, and age are independent predictors of stroke [75]. Anticoagulation has been associated with a 68% risk reduction in stroke in post-MI patients with LV thrombus and is now recommended for 3 months where LV thrombus formation post-MI occurs [76].

Trials evaluating the effectiveness of oral anticoagulation in post-MI patients have shown conflicting and inconclusive results. In a subgroup of patients with AF post-MI in the Efficacy and Safety of the oral direct Thrombin inhibitor ximElagatran in patients with rEcent Myocardial damage (ESTEEM) trial, 6.9% of patients treated with the combination of ximelagatran and aspirin had death, nonfatal MI, or stroke during a 6-month follow-up, compared with 20.6% of patients who received aspirin alone 0.30 (95% CI 0.12–0.74) [77]. The Coumadin Aspirin Reinfarction study (CARS) compared fixed low-dose warfarin (INR 1.3–1.8) with low-dose aspirin (80 mg daily) and found no difference in nonfatal reinfarction, nonfatal stroke or cardiovascular death (8.6% with aspirin versus 8.4% with warfarin) at a median of 14 months of follow-up [78]. Similar results were obtained in the Combination Haemotherapy and Mortality Prevention (CHAMP) trial [79]; this compared aspirin monotherapy with warfarin (mean INR 1.8) plus aspirin after acute MI, and found no differences in stroke (3.5% with aspirin and 3.1% with combination therapy) at a median 2.7-year follow-up.

By contrast, the Warfarin, Aspirin, Reinfarction (WARIS) II study [80] showed that anticoagulation with warfarin plus aspirin or with warfarin alone (within 4 weeks of MI) reduced a composite of mortality, nonfatal reinfarction, or stroke compared with aspirin alone (15% versus 16.7% versus 20%, respectively). There was an overall risk reduction of 29% with combination therapy and 19% with warfarin compared with aspirin alone at a median follow-up of 2.7 years, but at the expense of more hemorrhagic events in the warfarin groups (0.62% [warfarin groups] versus 0.17% [aspirin alone] per treatment year). The Antithrombotics in the Secondary Prevention of Events in Coronary Thrombosis-2 (ASPECT-2) study showed similar benefits of oral anticoagulation compared with antiplatelet therapy; there was a reduction in mortality, MI, and strokes (9% aspirin versus 5% warfarin versus 5% warfarin plus aspirin), but with a trend towards a higher hemorrhage rate with warfarin [81].

Nonetheless, there is still no clear consensus as to whether anticoagulant treatment of the whole cohort of patients with acute MI in sinus rhythm is more effective compared with conventional treatment with antiplatelets in reducing adverse cardiac events and, if it is, how long the treatment should continue.

A proportion (6–8%) of subjects presenting with ACS have pre-existing indications for long-term oral anticoagulation, for example, due to AF, mechanical heart valves, or VTE. Oral anticoagulation in ACS settings potentially poses several problems, which need to be considered. For example, triple therapy (two antiplatelet agents plus warfarin) tend to be associated with a higher risk of bleeding complications. Interruption of VKA therapy may expose the patient to an increased risk of thromboembolic episodes.

Accordingly, several precautions should be considered. Bare metal stents should be used, while usage of drug-eluting stents should be restricted to clinical and/or anatomical conditions, where their benefits are clearly established (eg, long lesions, small vessels, diabetes). Radial access should be the preferred choice in order to reduce the risk of periprocedural bleeding, particularly when repeated interventions are needed. Percutaneous coronary interventions without interruption of warfarin are generally preferred to avoid bridging therapy, which may increase the risk of bleeding or ischemic events.

Nevertheless, triple therapy (warfarin, aspirin, and clopidogrel) seems to have an acceptable risk–benefit ratio and should be used in the initial 3–6 months (or for longer in some patients at low-bleeding risk) [51]. ST segment elevation myocardial infarction (STEMI) and non-ST segment elevation myocardial infarction (NSTEMI) patients with a high-risk of cardiovascular thrombotic complications should be followed with a prolonged (up to 12 months) therapy of warfarin plus clopidogrel 75 mg daily (or, alternatively, aspirin 75–100 mg daily, plus gastric protection) [52,82].

Heart failure

Heart failure is an increasingly common condition and is associated with increased thromboembolic risk; however, the utility of chronic anticoagulant therapy in patients with heart failure is still controversial. The authors of a Cochrane systematic review of antithrombotic drugs in patients with heart failure found no robust evidence for additional benefits of anticoagulation over administration of aspirin in reducing mortality and thromboembolism [83,84]. Of note, hospitalizations were more common in aspirin users than in those managed with warfarin.

Possible benefits of long-term oral anticoagulation have been addressed in several trials (Table 2.9) [85,86]. For example, the Warfarin/ Aspirin Study in Heart failure (WASH) trial was a small pilot study that compared aspirin, warfarin, and no treatment in heart failure patients [85]. It found no statistical differences in the primary endpoint of death, nonfatal MI, or nonfatal stroke (26 [no treatment], 32 [aspirin], and 26% [warfarin]), after a mean follow up of 27 months. Nonetheless, the rate of hospitalization for worsening heart failure was significantly higher in the aspirin arm compared with the warfarin arm and the no-treatment arm ($P=0.044$ for warfarin versus aspirin).

Heart failure: summary of randomized clinical trials comparing warfarin and aspirin

Trials	Follow-up (months)	Head-to-head comparison	Results
WASH [85]	27	Warfarin (n=89) vs aspirin (n=91) vs no treatment (n=99)	No differences observed in primary outcomes (death or nonfatal MI or stroke) between treatment groups. More patients in aspirin group than warfarin group had CV-related hospitalizations or death (HR 1.39, 95% CI 0.95–2.00) during first 12 months of follow-up
WATCH [86]	18	Warfarin (n=540) vs aspirin (n=523) or clopidogrel (n=524)	No significant differences noted in primary outcomes (death or nonfatal MI or nonfatal strokes) between treatment groups. However, patients on aspirin had more heart failure related hospitalizations than those on warfarin ($P=0.019$)

Table 2.9 Heart failure: summary of randomized clinical trials comparing warfarin and aspirin. CI, confidence interval; CV, cardiovascular; HR, hazard ratio; MI, myocardial infarction; WASH, Warfarin/Aspirin Study in Heart failure; WATCH, Warfarin and Antiplatelet Therapy in Chronic Heart failure. Data from Cleland et al [85] and Massie et al [86].

Similar results were seen in the Warfarin and Antiplatelet Therapy in Chronic Heart failure (WATCH) trial in which patients with ejection fraction <35% were randomized to blinded antiplatelet therapy (aspirin or clopidogrel) or warfarin to prevent thromboembolic events [86]. In this study no difference was observed in the composite primary end-point of stroke, MI, or death (20.7% [aspirin] versus 21.6% [clopidogrel] versus 19.6% [warfarin]) at 18 months, follow-up. However, because of poor recruitment of patients, the study was terminated earlier than expected and therefore was underpowered.

The ongoing multicenter, double-blind, randomized Warfarin versus Aspirin with ReduCed Ejection Fraction (WARCEF) trial [87] is studying the benefits of warfarin or aspirin in heart failure patients and may provide evidence for the benefits of appropriate antithrombotic therapy in these patients.

Conclusions

Compelling evidence favors the use of appropriate antithrombotic thera-pies for the prevention of VTE as well as treatment of patients with VTE, AF, and implantation of prosthetic valves, and the range of indications for anticoagulant therapy may expand further. However, despite this, each patient who might require anticoagulation should be individu-ally assessed in terms of the potential benefits and risks of the therapy. Furthermore, the approach towards treatment needs to be holistic, and success is largely based on appropriate patient education to facilitate safer and effective use of anticoagulant therapies.

References

1   Heit JA, Melton LJ 3rd, Lohse CM, et al. Incidence of venous thromboembolism in hospitalized patients vs community residents. *Mayo Clin Proc*. 2001;76:1102-1110.
2   Fowkes FJ, Price JF, Fowkes FG. Incidence of diagnosed deep vein thrombosis in the general population: systematic review. *Eur J Vasc Endovasc Surg*. 2003;25:1-5.
3   Hansson PO, Sörbo J, Eriksson H. Recurrent venous thromboembolism after deep vein thrombosis: incidence and risk factors. *Arch Intern Med*. 2000;160:769-774.
4   Oger E. Incidence of venous thromboembolism: a community-based study in Western France. EPI-GETBP Study Group. Groupe d'Etude de la Thrombose de Bretagne Occidentale. Thromb Haemost. 2000;83:657-660.
5   Nordstrom M, Lindblad B. Autopsy-verified venous thromboembolism within a defined urban population - the city of Malmo, Sweden. APMIS. 1998;106:378-384.

6 Morrell MT, Dunnill MS. The post-mortem incidence of pulmonary embolism in a hospital population. *Br J Surg.* 1968;55:347-352.

7 Heit JA, Silverstein MD, Mohr DN, et al. Predictors of survival after deep vein thrombosis and pulmonary embolism: a population-based, cohort study. *Arch Intern Med.* 1999;159:445-453.

8 Agnelli G. Prevention of venous thromboembolism in surgical patients. Circulation. 2004;110:IV-4-IV-12.

9 Dentali F, Douketis JD, Gianni M, et al. Meta-analysis: anticoagulant prophylaxis to prevent symptomatic venous thromboembolism in hospitalized medical patients. *Ann Intern Med.* 2007;146:278-288.

10 Collins R, Scrimgeour A, Yusuf S, Peto R. Reduction in fatal pulmonary embolism and venous thrombosis by perioperative administration of subcutaneous heparin. Overview of results of randomized trials in general, orthopedic, and urologic surgery. *N Engl J Med.* 1988;318:1162-1173.

11 Clagett GP, Reisch JS. Prevention of venous thromboembolism in general surgical patients: results of meta-analysis. *Ann Surg.* 1988;208:227-240.

12 Mismetti P, Laporte S, Darmon JY, et al. Meta-analysis of low molecular weight heparin in the prevention of venous thromboembolism in general surgery. *Br J Surg.* 2001;88:913-930.

13 Wein L, Wein S, Haas SJ, et al. Pharmacological venous thromboembolism prophylaxis in hospitalized medical patients: a meta-analysis of randomized controlled trials. *Arch Intern Med.* 2007;167:1476-1486.

14 Deitelzweig SB, Becker R, Lin J, Benner J. Comparison of the two-year outcomes and costs of prophylaxis in medical patients at risk of venous thromboembolism. *Thromb Haemost.* 2008;100:810-820.

15 Nurmohamed MT, Rosendaal FR, Büller HR, et al. Low-molecular-weight heparin versus standard heparin in general and orthopaedic surgery: a meta-analysis. *Lancet.* 1992;340:152-156.

16 Hull RD, Raskob GE, Pineo G, et al. A comparison of subcutaneous low-molecular-weight heparin with warfarin sodium for prophylaxis against deep-vein thrombosis after hip or knee implantation. *N Engl J Med.* 1993;329:1370-1376.

17 Francis CW, Pellegrini VD Jr, Totterman S, et al. Prevention of deep-vein thrombosis after total hip arthroplasty. Comparison of warfarin and dalteparin. *J Bone Joint Surg Am.* 1997;79:1365-1372.

18 Agnelli, G, Bergqvist, D, Cohen A, Gallus AS, Gent M; PEGASUS investigators. Randomized clinical trial of postoperative fondaparinux versus perioperative dalteparin for prevention of venous thromboembolism in high-risk abdominal surgery. *Br J Surg.* 2005;92:1212-1220.

19 Francis CW, Berkowitz SD, Comp PC, et al; EXULT A Study Group. Comparison of ximelagatran with warfarin for the prevention of venous thromboembolism after total knee replacement. *N Engl J Med.* 2003;349:1703-1712.

20 Colwell CW Jr, Berkowitz SD, Lieberman JR, et al; EXULT B Study Group. Oral direct thrombin inhibitor ximelagatran compared with warfarin for the prevention of venous thromboembolism after total knee arthroplasty. *J Bone Joint Surg Am.* 2005;87:2169-2177.

21 Guyatt GH, Akl EA, Crowther M, et al. Executive summary: antithrombotic therapy and prevention of thrombosis, 9th ed: American College of Chest Physicians Evidence-Based Clinical Practice Guidelines. *Chest.* 2012;141;7S-47S.

22 Handoll HH, Farrar MJ, McBirnie J, et al. Heparin, low molecular weight heparin and physical methods for preventing deep vein thrombosis and pulmonary embolism following surgery for hip fractures. *Cochrane Database Syst Rev.* 2002;CD000305.

23 Dolovich LR, Ginsberg JS, Douketis JD, et al. A meta-analysis comparing low-molecular-weight heparins with unfractionated heparin in the treatment of venous thromboembolism: examining some unanswered questions regarding location of treatment, product type, and dosing frequency. *Arch Intern Med.* 2000;160:181-188.

24 Quinlan DJ, McQuillan A, Eikelboom JW. Low-molecular-weight heparin compared with intravenous unfractionated heparin for treatment of pulmonary embolism: a meta-analysis of randomized, controlled trials. *Ann Intern Med.* 2004;140:175-183.

25 Wilbur K, Lynd LD, Sadatsafavi M. Low-molecular-weight heparin versus unfractionated heparin for prophylaxis of venous thromboembolism in medicine patients–a pharmacoeconomic analysis. *Clin Appl Thromb Hemost.* 2011;17:454-465.

26 Vinson DR, Berman DA. Outpatient treatment of deep venous thrombosis: a clinical care pathway managed by the emergency department. *Ann Emerg Med.* 2001;37:251-258.

27 Smith BJ, Weekley JS, Pilotto L, et al. Cost comparison of at-home treatment of deep venous thrombosis with low molecular weight heparin to inpatient treatment with unfractionated heparin. *Intern Med J.* 2002;32:29-34.

28 Segal JB, Streiff MB, Hofmann LV, et al. Management of venous thromboembolism: a systematic review for a practice guideline. *Ann Intern Med.* 2007;146:211-222.

29 Büller HR, Davidson BL, Decousus H, et al; Matisse Investigators. Fondaparinux or enoxaparin for the initial treatment of symptomatic deep venous thrombosis: a randomized trial. *Ann Intern Med.* 2004;140:867-873.

30 Das SK, Cohen AT, Edmondson RA, et al. Low-molecular-weight heparin versus warfarin for prevention of recurrent venous thromboembolism: a randomized trial. *World J Surg.* 1996;20:521-526.

31 Lee AY, Levine MN, Baker RI, et al; Randomized Comparison of Low-Molecular-Weight Heparin versus Oral Anticoagulant Therapy for the Prevention of Recurrent Venous Thromboembolism in Patients with Cancer (CLOT) Investigators. Low-molecular-weight heparin versus a coumarin for the prevention of recurrent venous thromboembolism in patients with cancer. *N Engl J Med.* 2003;349:146-153.

32 Agnelli G, Prandoni P, Santamaria MG, et al; Warfarin Optimal Duration Italian Trial Investigators. Three months versus one year of oral anticoagulant therapy for idiopathic deep venous thrombosis. Warfarin Optimal Duration Italian Trial Investigators. *N Engl J Med.* 2001;345:165-169.

33 Schulman S, Rhedin AS, Lindmarker P, et al. A comparison of six weeks with six months of oral anticoagulant therapy after a first episode of venous thromboembolism. Duration of Anticoagulation Trial Study Group. *N Engl J Med.* 1995;332:1661-1665.

34 Schulman S, Granqvist S, Holmström M, et al. The duration of oral anticoagulant therapy after a second episode of venous thromboembolism. The Duration of Anticoagulation Trial Study Group. *N Engl J Med.* 1997;336:393-398.

35 Kearon C, Ginsberg JS, Kovacs MJ, et al; Extended Low-Intensity Anticoagulation for Thrombo-Embolism Investigators. Comparison of low-intensity warfarin therapy with conventional-intensity warfarin therapy for long-term prevention of recurrent venous thromboembolism. *N Engl J Med.* 2003;349:631-639.

36 Ridker PM, Goldhaber SZ, Danielson E, et al; PREVENT Investigators. Long-term, low-intensity warfarin therapy for the prevention of recurrent venous thromboembolism. *N Engl J Med.* 2003;348:1425-1434.

37 van Gogh Investigators; Buller HR, Cohen AT, et al. Idraparinux versus standard therapy for venous thromboembolic disease. *N Engl J Med.* 2007;357:1094-1104.

38 Elsharawy M, Elzayat E. Early results of thrombolysis vs anticoagulation in iliofemoral venous thrombosis. A randomised clinical trial. *Eur J Vasc Endovasc Surg.* 2002;24:209-214.

39 Comerota AJ, Throm RC, Mathias SD, et al. Catheter-directed thrombolysis for iliofemoral deep venous thrombosis improves health-related quality of life. *J Vasc Surg.* 2000;32:130-137.

40 Razavi MK, Wong H, Kee ST, et al. Initial clinical results of tenecteplase (TNK) in catheter-directed thrombolytic therapy. *J Endovasc Ther.* 2002;9:593-598.

41 Plate G, Einarsson E, Ohlin P, et al. Thrombectomy with temporary arteriovenous fistula: the treatment of choice in acute iliofemoral venous thrombosis. *J Vasc Surg.* 1984;1:867-876.

42 Decousus H, Leizorovicz A, Parent F, et al. A clinical trial of vena caval filters in the prevention of pulmonary embolism in patients with proximal deep-vein thrombosis. Prévention du Risque d'Embolie Pulmonaire par Interruption Cave Study Group. *N Engl J Med.* 1998;338:409-415.

43 White RH, Zhou H, Kim J, Romano PS. A population-based study of the effectiveness of inferior vena cava filter use among patients with venous thromboembolism. *Arch Intern Med.* 2000;160:2033-2041.

44 Wan S, Quinlan DJ, Agnelli G, Eikelboom JW. Thrombolysis compared with heparin for the initial treatment of pulmonary embolism: a meta-analysis of the randomized controlled trials. *Circulation.* 2004;110:744-749.

45 Keeling D, Baglin T, Tait C, et al; British Committee for Standards in Haematology. Guidelines on oral anticoagulation with warfarin - fourth edition. *Br J Haematol.* 2011;154:311-324.

46 Otten HM, Prins MH. Venous thromboembolism and occult malignancy. *Thromb Res.* 2001;102:V187-194.

47 Lloyd-Jones DM, Wang TJ, Leip EP, et al. Lifetime risk for development of atrial fibrillation: the Framingham heart study. *Circulation.* 2004;110:1042-1046.

48 Heeringa J, van der Kuip DA, Hofman A, et al. Prevalence, incidence and lifetime risk of atrial fibrillation: the Rotterdam study. *Eur Heart J.* 2006;27:949-953.

49 Stewart S, Hart CL, Hole DJ, McMurray JJ. Population prevalence, incidence, and predictors of atrial fibrillation in the Renfrew/Paisley study. *Heart.* 2001;86:516-521.

50 Miyasaka Y, Barnes ME, Gersh BJ, et al. Secular trends in incidence of atrial fibrillation in Olmsted County, Minnesota, 1980 to 2000, and implications on the projections for future prevalence. *Circulation.* 2006;114:119-125.

51 Camm AJ, Kirchhof P, Lip GY, et al. Guidelines for the management of atrial fibrillation: the Task Force for the Management of Atrial Fibrillation of the European Society of Cardiology (ESC). *Eur Heart J.* 2010;31:2369-2429.

52 Camm AJ, Kirchhof P, Lip GYH, et al; The Task Force for the Management of Atrial Fibrillation of the European Society of Cardiology (ESC). Guidelines for the management of atrial fibrillation. *Euro Heart J.* 2010;31:2369-2429.

53 Klein AL, Jasper SE, Katz WE, et al; ACUTE II Steering and Publications Committee for the ACUTE II Investigators. The use of enoxaparin compared with unfractionated heparin for short-term antithrombotic therapy in atrial fibrillation patients undergoing transoesophageal echocardiography-guided cardioversion: assessment of Cardioversion Using Transoesophageal Echocardiography (ACUTE) II randomized multicentre study. *Eur Heart J.* 2006;27:2858-65.

54 Wu LA, Chandrasekaran K, Friedman PA, et al. Safety of expedited anticoagulation in patients undergoing transesophageal echocardiographic-guided cardioversion. *Am J Med.* 2006;119:142-146.

55 Petersen P, Boysen G, Godtfredsen J, et al. Placebo-controlled, randomised trial of warfarin and aspirin for prevention of thromboembolic complications in chronic atrial fibrillation. The Copenhagen AFASAK study. *Lancet.* 1989;i:175-179.

56 Lip GY, Nieuwlaat R, Pisters R, Lane DA, Crijns HJ. Refining clinical risk stratification for predicting stroke and thromboembolism in atrial fibrillation using a novel risk factor-based approach: the euro heart survey on atrial fibrillation. *Chest.* 2010;137:263-72.

57 The Boston Area Anticoagulation Trial for Atrial Fibrillation Investigators. The effect of low-dose warfarin on the risk of stroke in patients with nonrheumatic atrial fibrillation. *N Engl J Med.* 1990;323:1505-1511.

58 Connolly SJ, Laupacis A, Gent M, et al. Canadian Atrial Fibrillation Anticoagulation (CAFA) Study. *J Am Coll Cardiol.* 1991;18:349-355.

59 EAFT (European Atrial Fibrillation Trial) Study Group. Secondary prevention in non-rheumatic atrial fibrillation after transient ischaemic attack or minor stroke. *Lancet.* 1993;342:1255-1262.

60 Stroke Prevention in Atrial Fibrillation Study. Final results. *Circulation.* 1991;84:527-539.

61 Ezekowitz MD, Bridgers SL, James KE, et al. Warfarin in the prevention of stroke associated with nonrheumatic atrial fibrillation. Veterans Affairs Stroke Prevention in Nonrheumatic Atrial Fibrillation Investigators. *N Engl J Med.* 1992;327:1406-1412.

62 Hart RG, Pearce LA, Agullar MI. Antithrombotic therapy to prevent stroke in patients who have nonvalvular atrial fibrillation: a meta-analysis. *Ann Intern Med.* 2007;146:857-867.

63 Lip GY, Edwards SJ. Stroke prevention with aspirin, warfarin and ximelagatran in patients with non-valvular atrial fibrillation: a systemic review and meta-analysis. *Thromb Res.* 2006;118:321-33.

64 Diener HC, Cunha L, Forbes C, et al. European Stroke Prevention Study. 2. Dipyridamole and acetylsalicylic acid in the secondary prevention of stroke. *J Neurol Sci.* 1996;143:1-13.

65 UK-TIA Study Group. The United Kingdom Transient Ischemic Attack (UK-TIA) aspirin trial: final results. *J Neurol Neurosurg Psychiatry.* 1991;54:1044-1054.

66 Japan Atrial Fibrillation Stroke Trial Group. Low-dose aspirin for prevention of stroke in low-risk patients with atrial fibrillation: Japan Atrial Fibrillation Stoke Trial. *Stroke.* 2006;37:447-451.

67 Posada IS, Barriales V. Alternate-day dosing of aspirin in atrial fibrillation. LASAF Pilot Study Group. *Am Heart J.* 1999;138:137-143.

68 Stroke Prevention in Atrial Fibrillation investigators. A differential effect of aspirin in prevention of stroke on atrial fibrillation. *J Stroke Cerebrovasc Dis.* 1993;3:181-188.

69 ACTIVE Writing Group on behalf of the ACTIVE Investigators. Clopidogrel plus aspirin versus oral anticoagulation for atrial fibrillation in the atrial fibrillation clopidogrel trial with irbesartan for prevention of vascular events (ACTIVE W). *Lancet.* 2006;367:1903-1912.

70 Mant J, Hobbs FD, Fletcher K, et al; BAFTA investigators; Midland Research Practices Network (MidReC). Warfarin versus aspirin for stroke prevention in an elderly community population with atrial fibrillation (the Birmingham Atrial Fibrillation Treatment of the Aged Study, BAFTA): a randomised controlled trial. *Lancet.* 2007;370:493-503.

71 Stein PD, Alpert JS, Bussey HI, et al. Antithrombotic therapy in patients with mechanical and biological prosthetic heart valves. *Chest.* 2001;119:220-227S.

72 American College of Cardiology/American Heart Association Task Force on Practice Guidelines; Society of Cardiovascular Anesthesiologists; Society for Cardiovascular Angiography and Interventions; Society of Thoracic Surgeons; Bonow RO, Carabello BA, Kanu C, et al. ACC/AHA 2006 guidelines for the management of patients with valvular heart disease: a report of the American College of Cardiology/American Heart Association Task Force on Practice Guidelines (writing committee to revise the 1998 Guidelines for the Management of Patients With Valvular Heart Disease): developed in collaboration with the Society of Cardiovascular Anesthesiologists: endorsed by the Society for Cardiovascular Angiography and Interventions and the Society of Thoracic Surgeons. *Circulation.* 2006;114:e84-231.

73 Vahanian A, Alfieri O, Andreotti F, et al; ESC Committee for Practice Guidelines. Guidelines on the management of valvular heart disease (version 2012): the Joint Task Force on the Management of Valvular Heart Disease of the European Society of Cardiology (ESC) and the European Association for Cardio-Thoracic Surgery (EACTS). *Eur Heart J.* 2012;33:2451-496.

74 Vaitkus PT. Left ventricular mural thrombus and the risk of embolic stroke after acute myocardial infarction. *J Cardiovasc Risk.* 1995;2:103-106.

75 Loh E, Sutton MS, Wun CC, et al. Ventricular dysfunction and the risk of stroke after myocardial infarction. *N Engl J Med.* 1997;336:251-257.

76 Antman EM, Anbe DT, Armstrong PW, et al. ACC/AHA Guidelines for the Management of Patients With ST-Elevation Myocardial Infarction – Executive summary: a report of the American College of Cardiology/American Heart Association Task Force on Practice Guidelines (Writing Committee to Revise the 1999 Guidelines for the Management of Patients with Acute Myocardial Infarction). *Circulation.* 2004;110:588-636.

77 Tangelder MJ, Frison L, Weaver D, et al. Effect of ximelagatran on ischemic events and death in patients with atrial fibrillation after acute myocardial infarction in the efficacy and safety of the oral direct thrombin inhibitor ximelagatran in patients with recent myocardial damage (ESTEEM) trial. *Am Heart J.* 2008;155:382-387.

78 Coumadin Aspirin Refarction Study (CARS) Investigators. Randomised double-blind trial of fixed low dose warfarin with aspirin after myocardial infarction. *Lancet.* 1997;350:389-396.

79 Fiore L, Ezekowitz MD, Brophy MT, et al. Department of Veterans Affairs Cooperative Studies Program Clinical Trial comparing combined warfarin and aspirin with aspirin alone in survivors of acute myocardial infarction: primary results of the CHAMP study. *Circulation.* 2002;105:557-563.

80 Hurlen M, Abdelnoor M, Smith P, et al. Warfarin, aspirin or both after myocardial infarction. *N Engl J Med.* 2002;347:969-974.

81 Van Es RF, Jonker JJC, Verheugt FWA, et al. Aspirin and coumadin after acute coronary syndromes (the ASPECT-2 study). *Lancet.* 2002;360:109-113.

82 Hamm CW, Bassand JP, Agewall S, et al. ESC Guidelines for the management of acute coronary syndromes in patients presenting without persistent ST-segment elevation: The Task Force for the management of acute coronary syndromes (ACS) in patients presenting without persistent ST-segment elevation of the European Society of Cardiology (ESC). *Eur Heart J.* 2011;32:2999-3054.

83 Lip GY, Gibbs CR. Antiplatelet agents versus control or anticoagulation for heart failure in sinus rhythm: a Cochrane systematic review. *Q J Med.* 2002;95:461-468.

84 Lip GYH, Gibbs CR. Anticoagulation for heart failure in sinus rhythm: a Cochrane systemic review. *Q J Med.* 2002;95:451-459.

85 Cleland JG, Findlay I, Jafri S, et al. The Warfarin/Aspirin Study in Heart Failure (WASH): a randomised trial comparing antithrombotic strategies for patients with heart failure. *Am Heart J.* 2004;148:157-164.

86 Massie BM. Randomized trial of warfarin, aspirin, and clopidogrel in patients with chronic heart failure: the Warfarin and Antiplatelet Therapy in Chronic Heart Failure (WATCH) trial. *Circulation.* 2009;119:1616-1624.

87 Warfarin versus Aspirin in Reduced Cardiac Ejection Fraction (WARCEF). www.clinicaltrials.gov/ct2/show/NCT00041938. ClinicalTrails.gov, A service of the U.S. National Institutes of Health. Updated August 16, 2011. Accessed July 13, 2013.

Chapter 3

Vitamin K antagonists and their limitations

Chee W Khoo, Eduard Shantsila, Gregory YH Lip

The vitamin K antagonists (VKAs) have been the mainstay of oral anti-coagulant therapy for more than 50 years, warfarin being the VKA most commonly used worldwide. The longstanding popularity of the VKAs is largely based on their effectiveness in the prevention and treatment of venous thromboembolism (VTE), as well as the prevention of systemic embolism in patients who have mechanical heart valves or atrial fibrillation (AF).

Pharmacology of warfarin

The pharmacological effects of warfarin are based on its ability to inhibit the activity of vitamin K-dependent coagulation factors (factors II, VII, IX, and X). To express their procoagulant activity these factors require γ-carboxylation, a process dependent on the availability of vitamin K, which in turn depends on normal functioning of the enzyme vitamin K epoxide reductase. Inhibition of this enzyme by warfarin causes a lack of vitamin K and consequently results in the production of functionally impaired, partially carboxylated and decarboxylated factors, with corresponding anticoagulant effects [1]. As well as their anticoagulant effect, VKAs also have procoagulant potential via prevention of carboxylation of anticoagulant proteins C and S. However, as a rule, the anticoagulation effects of VKAs outweigh their procoagulant properties.

G. Y. H. Lip and E. Shantsila (eds.), *Handbook of Oral Anticoagulation*, DOI: 10.1007/978-1-908517-96-8_3, © Springer Healthcare 2013

Warfarin consists of a racemic mixture of two optically active isomers, the R and S forms. The S-isomer is five-times more potent than the R-isomer with respect to vitamin K antagonism [2].

There is substantial variability in the oral absorption and bioavailability of warfarin due to its multiple interactions with dietary constituents, lifestyle factors, and concomitant drugs. For example, the administration of low-dose vitamin K can reverse the effect of warfarin, whereas high concentrations of vitamin K may result in its accumulation in the liver and make the patient resistant to warfarin for a prolonged period of time. Genetic factors also play a role in a patient's response to warfarin. Because of the interplay of all these characteristics, substantial inter- and intra-individual variability in dosing is typical of VKAs.

Warfarin is mainly bound to albumin in the plasma and metabolized by the liver. It has a relatively long half-life of approximately 40 hours. This means it often takes several days to reach therapeutic levels of the drug. Table 3.1 summarizes its main pharmacological characteristics.

Pharmacogenetics of warfarin

Polymorphisms of two genes, cytochrome P-450 enzyme 2C9 (*CYP450 2C9*) and vitamin K epoxide reductase complex 1 (*VKORC1*), have been identified as playing major roles in warfarin activity. *CYP450 2C9* is involved in the oxidative metabolism of the potent S-isomer of warfarin [3], and

Pharmacological characteristics of warfarin	
Target on coagulation cascade	**Vitamin K episode reductase**
Prodrug	No
Dosing	Variable
Bioavailability	Variable
Time to peak drug level	Variable
Half-life	40 hours
Route of elimination	Metabolisation in liver
Renal clearance	0%
Interaction	Polypharmacy, dietary vitamin K
Safety in pregnancy	No
Antidote	Vitamin K

Table 3.1 Pharmacological characteristics of warfarin.

mutations are independently associated with an abnormal response to warfarin. *CYP450 2C9* polymorphism explains approximately 10% of the variation in warfarin dosing among white Europeans, and it is relatively rare in Asian and African American populations [4].

Approximately 25% of the dosing variation between individuals is attributable to polymorphisms in *VKORC1*, the warfarin target gene [5]. Two main haplotypes were identified in a North American study: low-dose haplotype group A and high-dose haplotype group B [6]. In patients with the group A haplotype, which was relatively common in Asian-Americans, there was a more rapid achievement of the therapeutic range. In contrast, patients with group B haplotype, the prevalence of which was relatively high in the African-American population, were relatively resistant to warfarin.

Interactions of warfarin with other drugs and food

Various commonly used medications, diets, and comorbidities have been shown to interact with warfarin, accounting for much of the inter- and intra-individual variability in therapeutic dosing.

The drugs known to interact with warfarin are mainly inducers and inhibitors of *CYP450 2C9* [7], an enzyme responsible for the metabolism of the potent *S*-isomer of warfarin. *CYP450 2C9* inhibitors include amiodarone, fluconazole, isoniazid, and sertraline. Rifampicin and barbiturates are known to induce *CYP450 2C9*. Other enzymes, such as CYP1A2 and CYP3A4, are responsible for the metabolism of the *R*-isomer. Quinolones, macrolides, metronidazole, and fluconazole inhibit these enzymes. Commonly used drugs that inhibit liver enzymes and potentiate the effect of warfarin are summarized in Table 3.2. Commonly used drugs that induce liver enzymes and inhibit the effect of warfarin are summarized in Table 3.3.

Interactions of other drugs with warfarin relate to serum protein binding. Warfarin is highly protein bound in the serum and other highly protein-bound drugs can displace warfarin from serum albumin and potentiate its anticoagulant effect [8].

Foods that contain a high level of vitamin K, for example broccoli, reduce the effect of warfarin. Excessive use of alcohol, which interferes with liver enzymes, may also affect the metabolism of warfarin [7].

Drugs with enzyme-inhibiting properties that enhance warfarin's effects

Anti-infective	Cardiovascular	Others
Ciprofloxacin	Amiodarone	Citalopram
Erythromycin	Diltiazem	Sertraline
Co-trimoxazole	Fenofibrate	Entacapone
Fluconazole	Propafenone	Alcohol
Isoniazid	Propranolol	Disulfiram
Metronidazole	Quinidine	Phenytoin
Miconazole		Cimetidine

Table 3.2 Drugs with enzyme-inhibiting properties that enhance warfarin's effects.

Drugs with enzyme-inducing properties that inhibit warfarin's effects

Anti-infective	Central nervous system	Others
Rifampicin	Barbiturates	Mercaptopurine
Ribavirin	Carbamazepine	Mesalazine
	Chlordiazepoxide	Azathioprine

Table 3.3 Drugs with enzyme-inducing properties that inhibit warfarin's effects.

Additionally, some herbs have been found to modify the effects of warfarin; for example, St John's wort (used for treatment of depression) may reduce the anticoagulant effect [7].

Commencement of anticoagulation

Following administration of warfarin, newly synthesized, dysfunctional, vitamin K-dependent clotting factors gradually replace the normal clotting factors; however, the rate of replacement of each of the different factors varies substantially, and the full anticoagulant effect of warfarin is often delayed. Importantly, as well as being time-dependent, this effect also depends on the dose administered. Of note, it has occasionally been reported that prompt loading with high doses of warfarin may trigger blockade of the anticoagulant proteins C and S before the inhibition of coagulation factors commences, thus causing a brief and transitional rise in prothrombotic risk. However, the clinical relevance of this phenomenon has not been established and a slow-loading regimen may be safer for patients who do not require rapid anticoagulation.

The majority of patients achieve therapeutic anticoagulation within 3 or 4 days [9,10]. If rapid anticoagulation is needed, a higher loading dose of warfarin or concomitant heparin injections can be used, accompanied by daily monitoring of the international normalized ratio (INR).

Monitoring of warfarin therapy
Prothrombin time and international normalized ratio

The large number of pharmacological interactions of warfarin and the risk of severe hemorrhagic complications mandate thorough monitoring of its anticoagulant activity. Prothrombin time (PT) used to be the most common test used to monitor VKAs; however, PT reporting could not be standardized because it was measured using reagents that had variable sensitivity. The results were expressed in seconds or as a simple ratio of patient:normal PT. The results were often not comparable between different laboratories, and this led to confusion regarding the appropriate therapeutic range and dose of warfarin.

A better calibrated model, the INR, was adopted in 1982 [11]. The INR is the ratio of measured PT over mean normal PT, using a specific reagent of known sensitivity. INR is more reliable than the unconverted PT ratio [12]; hence, it is recommended for use in the initiation and monitoring of warfarin therapy. The recommended targets of INR for oral anticoagulant therapy have been well studied and are summarized in Table 3.4 [9].

In clinical practice, a therapeutic range is often used rather than a single target because the INR is highly variable. Thus, a target INR of 2.5 implies a therapeutic range of 2.0–3.0, whereas a target INR of 3.0 signifies a therapeutic range of 2.5–3.5.

The effectiveness and safety of warfarin are critically dependent on maintaining the INR within the therapeutic range. In order to achieve this, a monitoring system has to be in place.

Approaches to international normalized ratio monitoring

The traditional model of care for patients who take oral anticoagulants requires regular attendance at an anticoagulation clinic for INR monitoring. This service usually requires input from a physician, pathologist, specialist nurse, or even a pharmacist. A venous blood sample or capillary blood sample is used. If the INR result cannot be reported immediately,

Indications for oral anticoagulation and target international normalized ratio

Indication	Target INR
PE	2.5
DVT	2.5
Recurrence PE/DVT when not on warfarin	2.5
Recurrence PE/DVT when on warfarin	3.5
Nonvalvular atrial fibrillation	2.5
Electrical cardioversion	2.5
Symptomatic inherited thrombophilia	2.5
Mural thrombus	2.5
Cardiomyopathy	2.5
Aortic mechanical heart valve	2.5–3.5*
Mitral mechanical heart valve	3.0–3.5*

Table 3.4 Indications for oral anticoagulation and target international normalized ratio.
*Depending on types of valve implanted. DVT, deep vein thrombosis; INR, international normalized ratio; PE, pulmonary embolism.

the patient receives dosing and recall advice through the mail or by telephone. If the INR result is available when the patient is present a dosing recommendation can be made and the patient can be given a date for his or her next appointment. This cycle is continued for as long as the patient needs anticoagulation.

Some general practices have set up anticoagulation services in the community. They either obtain a venous sample and then make dosing recommendations and give recall advice once the INR result becomes available, or they use 'near-patient' or 'point-of-care' testing, with or without computer-assisted dosing.

An increasing number of patients are using near-patient or point-of-care coagulation monitoring devices for self-monitoring of long-term oral anticoagulant therapy. According to the recent meta-analysis of 11 trials with data for 6417 participants and 12,800 person-years of follow-up [13], self-monitoring of anticoagulation by subjects with AF was associated with a significant reduction in thromboembolic events (hazard ratio [HR] 0.51, 95% confidence interval [CI] 0.31–0.85), but not for major hemorrhagic events (HR 0.88, 0.74–1.06) or death (HR 0.82,

0.62–1.09). Of note, patients younger than age 55 years showed a very prominent decrease in thrombotic events (HR 0.33, 95% CI 0.17–0.66), as well as subjects with mechanical heart valve (HR 0.52, 0.35–0.77). Moreover, the approach was also manageable and safe in a subgroup of very elderly (≥85 years old) participants. The analysis showed that self-monitoring and self-management of oral coagulation is a safe option for suitable patients of all ages. Patients should also be offered the option to self-manage their disease with suitable healthcare support as back-up. Self-monitoring of INR provides an alternative to clinic-based monitoring; however, it requires appropriate infrastructure within the healthcare system to support the service.

INR monitoring is a difficult task, partly due to the high variability and narrow therapeutic window. One study conducted in a university teaching hospital and involving 2223 patients with AF showed that almost a third of the treatment time and close to half of the INR readings were outside the therapeutic range [14].

It is not surprising that INR monitoring comprises a significant burden for healthcare systems. This might explain why oral anticoagulation therapy is still suboptimal despite well-publicized guidelines. There is physician reluctance to prescribe oral anticoagulation therapy, as reflected by the Euro Heart Survey finding that only 67% of patients eligible for the therapy were actually prescribed it [15]. This is discussed in more detail in Chapter 4.

Conclusions

Until recently, VKAs were the only choice for oral anticoagulation; warfarin being the most commonly used VKA worldwide. However, the utility of warfarin is limited by its narrow therapeutic window and slow onset and offset of action, as well as by substantial inter- and intra-individual variability in the therapeutic dose, which all necessitate regular dose adjustment to keep within the therapeutic range. Furthermore, the metabolism of warfarin is also influenced by genetic polymorphisms and by dietary and numerous drug interactions. All these factors have made INR monitoring a difficult task.

References

1   Malhotra OP, Nesheim ME, Mann KG. The kinetics of activation of normal and gamma carboxy glutamic acid deficient prothrombins. *J Biol Chem*. 1985;260:279-287.

2   Hirsh J, Fuster V, Ansell J, Halperin JL; American Heart Association/American College of Cardiology Foundation. American Heart Association/American College of Cardiology Foundation guide to warfarin therapy. *J Am Coll Cardiol*. 2003;41:1633-1652.

3   Mannucci PM. Genetic control of anticoagulation. *Lancet*. 1999;353:688-689.

4   Sanderson S, Emery J, Higgins J. CYP2C9 gene variants, drug dose, and bleeding risk in warfarin-treated patients: a HuGEnet systematic review and meta-analysis. *Genet Med*. 2005;7:97-104.

5   Wen MS, Lee M, Chen JJ, et al. Prospective study of warfarin dosage requirements based on CYP2C9 and VKORC1 genotypes. *Clin Pharmacol Ther*. 2008;84:83-89.

6   Rieder MJ, Reiner AP, Gage BF, et al. Effect of VKORC1 haplotypes on transcriptional regulation and warfarin dose. *N Engl J Med*. 2005;352:2285-2293.

7   Holbrook AM, Pereira JA, Labiris R, et al. Systematic overview of warfarin and its drug and food interaction. *Arch Intern Med*. 2005;165:1095-1106.

8   Gage BF, Fihn SD, White RH. Management and dosing of warfarin therapy. *Am J Med*. 2000;109:481-488.

9   Baglin TP, Keeling DM, Watson HG. Guidelines on oral anticoagulation (warfarin): third edition – 2005 update. *Br J Haematol*. 2006;132:277-285.

10 Hirsh J, Dalen J, Anderson DR, et al. Oral anticoagulants: mechanism of action, clinical effectiveness, and optimal therapeutic range. *Chest*. 2001;119(suppl):8-21S.

11 Kirkwood TBL. Calibration of reference thromboplastins and standardisation of the prothrombin time ratio. *Thromb Haemost*. 1983;49:238-244.

12 Johnston M, Harrison L, Moffat K, et al. Reliability of the international normalized ratio for monitoring the induction phase of warfarin: comparison with the prothrombin time ratio. *J Lab Clin Med*. 1996;128:214-217.

13 Heneghan C, Ward A, Perera R, et al. Self-monitoring of oral anticoagulation: systematic review and meta-analysis of individual patient data. *Lancet*. 2012;379:322-334.

14 Jones M, McEwan P, Morgan CL, et al. Evaluation of the pattern of treatment, level of anticoagulation control, and outcome of treatment with warfarin in patients with non-valvular atrial fibrillation: a record linkage study in a large British population. *Heart*. 2005;91:472-477.

15 Nieuwlaat R, Capucci A, Lip GY, et al; Euro Heart Survey Investigators. Antithrombotic treatment in real-life atrial fibrillation patients: a report from the Euro Heart Survey on Atrial Fibrillation. *Eur Heart J*. 2006;27:3018-3026.

Chapter 4

Hemorrhage risks, patient perspectives, and quality-of-life issues

Kok-Hoon Tay, Stavros Apostolakis, Deirdre A Lane,
Gregory YH Lip

Warfarin is a widely used medication, which is often prescribed to high-risk patients with multiple comorbidities who are receiving multiple medications and thus poses a risk of side-effects related to its pharmacologic properties and drug interactions. It is estimated that, in the UK, for example, 950,000 patients are currently taking warfarin (2% of the general practice population). This number is expected to rise by approximately 10% per annum, primarily because of its use in AF [1].

Commencing warfarin is not without its risks and complications. Warfarin has diverse pharmacokinetics and pharmacodynamics in different patients, which result in the need for individual dose-adjustment based on the international normalized ratio (INR). Monitoring to maintain anticoagulation within the therapeutic range is essential to minimize warfarin-related complications, such as hemorrhage or thromboembolic events. Furthermore, it is also required because warfarin's anticoagulant properties are affected by a number of medications (antibiotics, especially macrolides/quinolones, antifungals, anticonvulsants such as phenytoin, nonsteroidal anti-inflammatory drugs, and amiodarone) and by alcohol, herbal medicines, and foods high in vitamin K, as already discussed in Chapter 3.

G. Y. H. Lip and E. Shantsila (eds.), *Handbook of Oral Anticoagulation*, 41
DOI: 10.1007/978-1-908517-96-8_4, © Springer Healthcare 2013

In the absence of prospective data from 'real world' populations all available information on hemorrhagic risk associated with oral direct thrombin inhibitors and factor Xa inhibitors has been derived from phase III clinical trials. In these settings all new agents have demonstrated bleeding rates equal or lower than adjusted dose warfarin.

In the landmark Randomized Evaluation of Long-Term Anticoagulation Therapy (RE-LY) trial the direct thrombin inhibitor dabigatran 150 mg was superior to warfarin for the prevention of stroke or systemic embolism (1.11 versus 1.71 per 100 patient-years, $P<0.001$ for superiority); however, rates of major bleeding were similar in the two arms (3.32% versus 3.57% per year for dabigatran 150 mg [twice daily] and warfarin, respectively $P=0.32$) [2]. With respect to subtypes of major bleeding, rates of intracranial hemorrhage were lower in both dabigatran arms (110 mg or 150 mg twice daily), while major gastrointestinal bleeds were higher with dabigatran 150 mg twice daily compared both with warfarin and with dabigatran 110 mg twice daily. A post-hoc analysis of the RE-LY trial demonstrated that both doses of dabigatran compared with warfarin had lower risks of both intracranial and extracranial bleeding in patients aged <75 years. In the subgroup of patients aged ≥75 years, intracranial bleeding risk was lower but extracranial bleeding risk was similar or higher with both doses of dabigatran compared with warfarin [3].

In the Rivaroxaban Once Daily Oral Direct Factor Xa Inhibition Compared with Vitamin K Antagonism for Prevention of Stroke and Embolism Trial in Atrial Fibrillation (ROCKET-AF) trial, rivaroxaban was superior to warfarin in the as-treated population for the prevention of stroke or systemic embolism (1.7% versus 2.2% per year, $P<0.001$) [4]. There were no significant differences in the overall major bleedings between rivaroxaban and warfarin (3.6% versus 3.4% per year, $P=0.58$, respectively). Intracranial and fatal hemorrhages, however, were significantly reduced in the rivaroxaban arm (0.5% vs. 0.7%, $P=0.02$ and 0.2% vs. 0.5%, $P=0.003$, respectively), while major gastrointestinal bleedings were more frequent. A post-hoc analysis of the subgroup of patients with moderate renal impairment, who were treated with reduced dosage of rivaroxaban, provided results consistent with the overall trial [5].

In the Apixaban for Reduction in Stroke and Other Thromboembolic Events in Atrial Fibrillation (ARISTOTLE) study, apixaban was superior to warfarin in the primary outcome of stroke or systemic embolism. The relative risk reduction (RRR) in the primary endpoint was largely driven by a reduction in hemorrhagic stroke, with no significant difference in ischemic stroke rate between apixaban and warfarin. Rates of major bleeding events were lower in the apixaban group compared with warfarin (2.13% versus 3.09% per year, $P<0.001$), particularly intracranial hemorrhages [6]. Interestingly, in the Apixaban Versus Acetylsalicylic Acid to Prevent Strokes (AVERROES) study, apixaban was superior to aspirin in the primary outcome of stroke and systemic embolism and was associated with the reduction in the rate of death without increasing the risk of major bleeding (1.4% versus 1.2% per year, $P=0.57$) [7].

There is a multitude of physician- and patient-related factors that lead to underutilization of oral anticoagulant therapy, along with the risk of hemorrhage; these are discussed in the following sections.

Warfarin and risk of hemorrhage

The most common side-effect from warfarin is hemorrhage from any anatomical site. The most feared complication from over-anticoagulation (INR >3.0) is intracranial hemorrhage, which accounts for approximately 90% of deaths from warfarin-associated hemorrhage and for the majority of disability among survivors [8]. Moreover, the benefit of warfarin is only conferred upon atrial fibrillation (AF) patients if the minimum percentage of time spent within the therapeutic INR range is between 58% and 65% [9]. Given the inherent difficulties associated with warfarin control, initiating warfarin is not always a straightforward decision, especially in elderly patients in whom the situation is usually compounded by multiple comorbidities, which further increase the risk of hemorrhage.

Nonetheless, intracranial hemorrhage rates in clinical trials conducted in AF patients on oral anticoagulant therapy are low, reported to be between 0.3 and 0.6% per year [10], and the absolute increase in major extracranial hemorrhages is even smaller, at ≤0.3% per year [11]. It may be that these figures reflect better quality INR monitoring and greater intensity of intervention by anticoagulation services in clinical trials, and outside the research setting the actual figures may be higher.

However, as reported by Hart and collegues, with careful INR monitoring and dose adjustment of oral anticoagulant therapy, warfarin can significantly reduce the risk of cardioembolic stroke by 64% (95% confidence interval [CI] 49–74%) compared to placebo, and by 39% (95% CI 22–52%) compared with antiplatelet agents [12]. The risk of intracranial hemorrhage associated with warfarin use was twice that of aspirin but the absolute risk was small at 0.2% per year [12]. Furthermore, among elderly patients (>75 years), the rate of major hemorrhage in aspirin users (2.0% per year) does not differ significantly from warfarin users (1.9% per year), as evidenced by the Birmingham Atrial Fibrillation of the Aged (BAFTA) study [13].

Risk factors for hemorrhage

There are many risk factors that increase the risk of hemorrhage in patients on oral anticoagulant therapy, such as:

- increasing age (≥60 years);
- previous stroke; and
- comorbidities, ie, diabetes mellitus, recent myocardial infarction, anemia (defined as hematocrit <30%), presence of malignancy, concomitant antiplatelet usage, uncontrolled hypertension, liver/renal failure, and previous gastrointestinal bleed.

Many of the risk factors for hemorrhage are also risk factors for stroke, and therefore the decision as to whether to commence oral anticoagulation should be highly individualized [14]. There are numerous stroke risk stratification schema to assist decision-making in prescribing oral anticoagulant therapy for AF patients, such as the CHADS2 (Congestive heart failure, Hypertension, Age >75, Diabetes mellitus and previous Stroke) schema, and other schemata from the American College of Cardiology (ACC), American College of Chest Physicians (ACCP), American Heart Association (AHA), European Society of Cardiology (ESC), and UK National Institute for Health and Clinical Excellence (NICE). By contrast, however, there is currently no universal hemorrhage risk stratification schema commonly employed in clinical practice.

To date, six hemorrhage risk predictor schemas have been proposed (Table 4.1) [15–21]. All six utilize age as one of the consistent predictors of hemorrhage risks, albeit with varying age categories: Kuijer et al [16] use age ≥60 years (lowest age), whereas Gage et al [18] use age >75 years (highest age). Only the Kuijer et al [16] and Shireman et al [17] models include female sex as a risk factor for hemorrhage when on warfarin. Previous significant hemorrhage and anemia (defined as hematocrit <30%) are regarded as important risk factors in all models [15,17–20] except that of Kuijer et al [16]. Other comorbid risk factors taken into account in the schemas include previous history of stroke, liver/renal failure, presence of diabetes mellitus, antiplatelet usage, uncontrolled hypertension, thrombocytopenia, excessive falls, alcohol abuse, and recent myocardial infarction.

Published hemorrhage risk schema

Study	Low	Moderate	High	Risk factors for score calculation
Beyth et al [15]	0	1–2	≥3	Age ≥65 years, gastrointestinal bleed in 2 weeks, previous stroke, comorbidities (1 of 4 – recent myocardial infarction, anemia, diabetes mellitus, and renal impairment), with 1 point for presence of each condition and 0 for absence
Kuijer et al [16]	0	1–3	>3	Risk score = (1.6 x age) + (1.3 x sex) + (2.2 x malignancy), with 1 point for being ≥60 years, female or presence of malignancy and 0 for absence
Shireman et al [17]	≤1.07	>1.07 but <2.19	≥2.19	Risk score = (0.49 x age) + (0.32 x female) + (0.58 x remote bleed) + (0.62 x recent bleed) + (0.71 x alcohol/drug abuse) + (0.27 x diabetes) + (0.86 x anemia) + (0.32 x antiplatelet), with 1 point for presence of each condition and 0 for absence
Gage et al [18]	0–1	2–3	≥4	Hepatic/renal disease, alcohol abuse, malignancy, older (age >75 years), ↓ platelet count, rebleeding risk, uncontrolled hypertension, anemia, genetic factor, excessive falls, stroke, with 2 points given to previous bleed and 1 point to each of the other factors
Pisters et al [19]	<3		≥3	Hypertension (uncontrolled), abnormal renal or liver function, stroke, previous bleeding, labile INR, age (>65 years), drugs, or alcohol. One point for each variable
Fang et al [20]	<4	4	>4	Anemia 3 points, severe renal disease 3 points, age ≥75 years 2 points, any prior hemorrhage 1 point, hypertension (diagnosed) 1 point

Table 4.1 Published hemorrhage risk schema. Data from [15–20]. Adapted and updated with permission from Tay et al [21]. © 2008 Schattauer GmbH.

Collectively, these six hemorrhage risk models were derived from studies of patients who were on warfarin for numerous reasons and not just for AF, for instance, including patients who had valvular heart surgery, deep vein thrombosis (DVT), pulmonary embolism (PE), stroke, transient ischemic attack, or other thromboembolism. The four most recent schemas [17–20] were drawn from populations consisting exclusively of AF patients. It is worth noting that these four hemorrhage risk predictor models were derived from mainly white populations, and the risk factors may not necessarily translate to nonwhite patients. Hence, there is very little consensus on the risk factors included within these schemas, and they lack clinical validation in an AF population. Consequently their predictive value is unknown, limiting their widespread clinical application [21].

Physician barriers to use of warfarin

Despite the wealth of evidence for the superiority of warfarin over aspirin in thromboprophylaxis to minimize stroke risk in AF (RRR 39%, 95% CI 22–52%) [12], the Euro Heart Survey demonstrated that only 67% of eligible AF patients are actually prescribed oral anticoagulant therapy [22]. Physicians' reluctance to prescribe warfarin is often due to a misperception of the magnitude of the risk of hemorrhage, overestimation of the associated risks, underestimation of the stroke risk, and clinical uncertainty or inexperience with warfarin [23]. Physicians who have more experience with warfarin or longer-standing practices tend to be more willing to prescribe it than their younger, less experienced counterparts [24,25].

A national survey conducted among Australian family physicians treating nonvalvular AF patients revealed that a higher percentage of the physicians reported a stroke in a patient who was not on an oral anticoagulant compared with those that reported an intracranial hemorrhage in a patient who was on an oral anticoagulant (45.8% versus 15.8%) [25]. Despite this, a physician's exposure to adverse events, such as hemorrhage, may play an exaggerated role in treatment decisions. Indeed, one study reported that adverse outcomes from anticoagulation have a greater influence on management decisions than occurrences of avoidable ischemic stroke: the odds of a physician prescribing warfarin were reduced after exposure to a patient who had serious hemorrhage when taking warfarin, but they were not changed after exposure to a patient who had thromboembolic event while not taking warfarin [26].

Patient barriers to use of warfarin

By contrast, patients are more concerned with reducing the risk of ischemic stroke [27]; hence, they are more accepting of warfarin and its inherent problems (life-long monitoring of INR, and interactions with food, alcohol, and drugs), and of the associated risk of hemorrhage, in order to avoid an ischemic stroke and its consequences [24].

Nevertheless, there are patient barriers to warfarin prescription, the most pertinent of which are patients' often limited knowledge about the disease, its treatment, the risk–benefit ratio of warfarin thromboprophylaxis [28], and their preferences for treatment [23]. It is important to involve patients in the decision-making process of whether or not to initiate warfarin [29]. Research has demonstrated that patients who are well-informed about treatment regimens are less anxious and more satisfied with treatment, and have higher rates of compliance and better outcomes [30]. Patient preferences for treatment need to be considered, given that the success of thromboprophylactic therapy and avoidance of warfarin-related complications rely largely on the patients' adherence to the warfarin regimen, complying with regular INR monitoring and taking into account drug, food, and alcohol interactions. A study of patients' preferences for anticoagulant treatment revealed that two out of five patients would prefer not to receive it, which may be due to misconceptions about anticoagulants and patients' lack of understanding of the reduction in stroke risk associated with anticoagulation [29]. A brief educational intervention demonstrated an improvement in patients' knowledge of AF and the need for anticoagulation, and the factors affecting INR control [31].

Quality of life in atrial fibrillation

As discussed in Chapter 2, warfarin remains the most widely used prophylaxis for AF patients who have at least moderate risk of stroke.

The development of AF in any patient and its subsequent treatment can encroach on aspects of patients' health-related quality of life (HRQoL). AF may give the impression of being a benign cardiac arrhythmia but it can be a disabling heart disease with complications related to the treatment strategy, be it 'rate control' or 'rhythm control,' which impact negatively on HRQoL.

There have been many studies conducted assessing the impact of interventional/noninterventional treatment strategies for rate/rhythm control on HRQoL in AF patients [32]. HRQoL is impaired in patients with AF compared with healthy controls [33]. It has been demonstrated that HRQoL can be significantly improved by either rate or rhythm control, but there does not appear to be a clear benefit of one treatment modality over the other in terms of HRQoL. Two randomized controlled trials AFFIRM (Atrial Fibrillation Follow-up Investigation of Rhythm Management) [34] and RACE (Rate Control Versus Electrical Cardioversion Study) [33] compared HRQoL directly for rate and rhythm strategies, rather than changes within each strategy from baseline. Both studies found no significant differences between rhythm and rate control in any of the HRQoL subscales on the Short Form-36 health survey questionnaires. However, most AF patients report a significant improvement in HRQoL after having had atrioventricular (AV) node ablation with or without pacing, radiofrequency catheter ablation/pulmonary vein isolation, and the Maze operation [32], which is probably due to the reduction in, or resolution of, symptoms following these interventions.

Another important consideration is the impact of oral anticoagulant therapy on HRQoL in AF patients. It appears that treatment strategy, 'rate or rhythm control,' exerts more influence over HRQoL than anti-coagulation therapy. A cross-sectional study conducted in 330 elderly (age >75 years) AF patients revealed that long-term warfarin (>1 year) itself did not affect their physical or mental HRQoL compared with the general elderly population [35]. Likewise, there is no change in HRQoL in a younger AF population (mean age 68 years) either, as demonstrated in the North American study, Boston Area Anticoagulation Trial for Atrial Fibrillation (BAATAF) [36].

Conclusions

When physicians are faced with a newly diagnosed AF patient, a wide spectrum of factors needs to be considered, in addition to management of the AF itself. Patients' perceptions about the disease and its treatment need to be assessed. Patients need to be encouraged to be active participants in their own healthcare. The success of treatment, of rate or rhythm control and of anticoagulation, requires patient adherence to a revised lifestyle regimen.

Currently, the complexities involved in managing warfarin treatment (regular INR checks, and awareness of drug, food, and alcohol interactions) mean that not all eligible patients are prescribed it, due to safety and compliance concerns. With the advent of novel anticoagulants, such as direct oral thrombin inhibitors (ie, dabigatran) or factor Xa inhibitors (apixaban, rivaroxaban, edoxaban), some of the inherent problems, such as regular INR monitoring and dose adjustment, and drug, food, and alcohol interactions, will be removed, hopefully enabling more eligible patients to receive oral anticoagulant therapy.

References

1   Connock M, Stevens C, Fry-Smith A, et al. Clinical effectiveness and cost-effectiveness of different models of managing long-term oral anticoagulation therapy: a systematic review and economic modeling. *Health Technol Assess*. 2007;11:iii-iv, ix-66.

2   Connolly SJ, Ezekowitz MD, Yusuf S, et al; RE-LY Steering Committee and Investigators. Dabigatran versus warfarin in patients with atrial fibrillation. *N Engl J Med*. 2009;361:1139-1151.

3   Eikelboom JW, Wallentin L, Connolly SJ, et al. Risk of bleeding with 2 doses of dabigatran compared with warfarin in older and younger patients with atrial fibrillation: an analysis of the randomized evaluation of long-term anticoagulant therapy (RE -LY) trial. *Circulation*. 2011;123:2363-2372.

4   Patel MR, Mahaffey KW, Garg J, et al; ROCKET AF Investigators. Rivaroxaban versus warfarin in nonvalvular atrial fibrillation. *N Engl J Med*. 2011;365:883-891.

5   Fox KA, Piccini JP, Wojdyla D, et al. Prevention of stroke and systemic embolism with rivaroxaban compared with warfarin in patients with non-valvular atrial fibrillation and moderate renal impairment. *Eur Heart J*. 2011;32:2387-2394.

6   Granger CB, Alexander JH, McMurray JJ, et al; ARISTOTLE Committees and Investigators. Apixaban versus warfarin in patients with atrial fibrillation. *N Engl J Med*. 2011;365:981-992.

7   Connolly SJ, Eikelboom J, Joyner C, et al; AVERROES Steering Committee and Investigators. Apixaban in patients with atrial fibrillation. *N Engl J Med*. 2011;364:806-817.

8   Fang MC, Go AS, Chang Y, et al. Death and disability from warfarin-associated intracranial and extracranial haemorrhages. *Am J Med*. 2007;120:700-705.

9   Connolly SJ, Pogue J, Eikelboom J, et al; ACTIVE W Investigators. Benefit of oral anticoagulant over antiplatelet therapy in atrial fibrillation depends on the quality of international normalized ratio control achieved by centers and countries as measured by time in therapeutic range. *Circulation.* 2008;118:2029-2037.

10 Hart RG, Tonarelli SB, Pearce LA. Avoiding central nervous system bleeding during antithrombotic therapy: recent data and ideas. *Stroke.* 2005;36:1588-1593.

11 Lip GY, Lim HS. Atrial fibrillation and stroke prevention. *Lancet Neurol.* 2007;6:981-993.

12 Hart RG, Pearce LA, Aguilar MI. Meta-analysis: antithrombotic therapy to prevent stroke in patients who have nonvalvular atrial fibrillation. *Ann Intern Med.* 2007;146:857-867.

13 Mant J, Hobbs FD, Fletcher K, et al; BAFTA investigators; Midland Research Practices Network (MidReC). Warfarin versus aspirin for stroke prevention in an elderly community population with atrial fibrillation (the Birmingham Atrial Fibrillation Treatment of the Aged Study, BAFTA): a randomised controlled trial. *Lancet.* 2007;370:493-503.

14 Poli D, Antonucci E, Marcucci R, et al. Risk of bleeding in very old atrial fibrillation patients on warfarin: relationship with ageing and CHADS2 score. *Thromb Res.* 2007;121:347-352.

15 Beyth RJ, Quinn LM, Landefeld CS. Prospective evaluation of an index for predicting the risk of major bleeding in outpatients treated with warfarin. *Am J Med.* 1998;105:91-99.

16 Kuijer PMM, Hutten BA, Prins MH, Büller HR. Prediction of the risk of bleeding during anticoagulant treatment for venous thromboembolism. *Arch Intern Med.* 1999;159:457-460.

17 Shireman TI, Mahnken JD, Howard PA, et al. Development of a contemporary bleeding risk model for elderly warfarin recipients. *Chest.* 2006;130:1390-1396.

18 Gage BF, Yan Y, Milligan PE, et al. Clinical classification schemes for predicting haemorrhage: Results from the National Registry of Atrial Fibrillation (NRAF). *Am Heart J.* 2006;151:713-719.

19 Pisters R, Lane DA, Nieuwlaat R, de Vos CB, Crijns HJ, Lip GY. A novel user-friendly score (HAS-BLED) to assess 1-year risk of major bleeding in patients with atrial fibrillation: the Euro Heart Survey. *Chest.* 2010;138:1093-1100.

20 Fang MC, Go AS, Chang Y, et al. A new risk scheme to predict warfarin-associated hemorrhage: the ATRIA (Anticoagulation and Risk Factors in Atrial Fibrillation) study. *J Am Coll Cardiol.* 2011;58:395-401.

21 Tay KH, Lane DA, Lip GY. Bleeding risks with combination of oral anticoagulation plus antiplatelet therapy: is clopidogrel any safer than aspirin when combined with warfarin? *Thromb Haemost.* 2008;100:955-957.

22 Nieuwlaat R, Capucci A, Lip GY, et al; Euro Heart Survey Investigators. Antithrombotic treatment in real-life atrial fibrillation patients: a report from the Euro Heart Survey on Atrial Fibrillation. *Eur Heart J.* 2006;27:3018-3026.

23 Lane DA, Lip GY. Barriers to anticoagulation in patients with atrial fibrillation: changing physician-related factors. *Stroke.* 2008;39:7-9.

24 Bungard TJ, Ghali WA, Teo KK, et al. Why do patients with atrial fibrillation not receive warfarin? *Arch Intern Med.* 2000;160:41-46.

25 Gattellari M, Worthington J, Zwar N, Middleton S. Barriers to the use of anticoagulation for nonvalvular atrial fibrillation: a representative survey of Australian family physicians. *Stroke.* 2008;39:227-230.

26 Choudhry NK, Anderson GM, Laupacis A, et al. Impact of adverse events on prescribing warfarin in patients with atrial fibrillation: matched pair analysis. *BMJ.* 2006;332:141-145.

27 Devereaux PJ, Anderson DR, Gardner MJ, et al. Differences between perspectives of physicians and patients on anticoagulation in patients with atrial fibrillation: observational study. *BMJ.* 2001;323:1218-1222.

28 Lip GY, Agnelli G, Thach AA, et al. Oral anticoagulation in atrial fibrillation: a pan-European patient survey. *Eur J Intern Med.* 2007;18:202-208.

29 Protheroe J, Fahey T, Montgomery AA, Peters TJ. The impact of patients' preferences on the treatment of atrial fibrillation: observational study of patient based decision analysis. *BMJ.* 2000;320:1380-1384.

30 Lane D, Lip GY. Anti-thrombotic therapy for atrial fibrillation and patients' preferences for treatment. *Age Ageing*. 2005;34:1-3.

31 Lane DA, Ponsford J, Shelley A, et al. Patient knowledge and perceptions of atrial fibrillation and anticoagulant therapy: effects of an educational intervention programme. The West Birmingham Atrial Fibrillation Project. *Int J Cardiol*. 2006;110:354-358.

32 Thrall G, Lane D, Carroll D, Lip GY. Quality of life in patients with atrial fibrillation: a systematic review. *Am J Med*. 2006;119:448.e1-19.

33 Hagens VE, Ranchor AV, Van Sonderen E, et al; RACE Study Group. Effect of rate or rhythm control on quality of life in persistent atrial fibrillation. Results from the Rate Control Versus Electrical Cardioversion (RACE) Study. *J Am Coll Cardiol*. 2004;43:241-247.

34 Jenkins LS, Brodsky M, Schron E, et al. Quality of life in atrial fibrillation: the Atrial Fibrillation Follow-up Investigation of Rhythm Management (AFFIRM) study. *Am Heart J*. 2005;149:112-120.

35 Das AK, Willcoxson PD, Corrado OJ, West RM. The impact of long-term warfarin on the quality of life of elderly people with atrial fibrillation. *Age Ageing*. 2007;36:95-97.

36 Lancaster TR, Singer DE, Sheehan MA, et al. The impact of long-term warfarin therapy on quality of life. Evidence from a randomized trial. Boston Area Anticoagulation Trial for Atrial Fibrillation Investigators. *Arch Intern Med*. 1991;151:1944-1949.

Chapter 5

New oral anticoagulants

Direct thrombin inhibitors

Eduard Shantsila, Stavros Apostolakis, Gregory YH Lip

Anticoagulation can be achieved by inhibition of the various coagulation factors. For example, as discussed in the preceding chapters, warfarin reduces the level of functional vitamin K-dependent factors II (prothrombin), VII, IX, and X by preventing their γ-carboxylation. Novel oral anticoagulant development has focused on the synthesis of selective inhibitors of coagulation factors, preferably acting independently of cofactors. The novel anticoagulants act on a number of targets in the coagulation cascade, but two of its key factors, Xa and IIa (thrombin), are the major therapeutic targets. As they are involved in the final steps of the coagulation cascade, their inhibition allows blocking of both intrinsic (plasma) and extrinsic (tissue) coagulation pathways.

Because the serine protease thrombin is the final mediator in the coagulation cascade that leads to the production of fibrin, the main protein component of blood clots [1], and is also a potent activator of platelets, it has been a popular target for the development of novel anticoagulants [2]. Several direct thrombin inhibitors (DTIs) have been approved for clinical use in the prevention of thrombosis, for example desirudin. However, these agents still require parenteral administration, limiting their chronic use, and the need for development of efficient, safe, convenient, and predictable oral anticoagulants remains.

G. Y. H. Lip and E. Shantsila (eds.), *Handbook of Oral Anticoagulation*, 53
DOI: 10.1007/978-1-908517-96-8_5, © Springer Healthcare 2013

Historical excursus: ximelagatran

Ximelagatran, a prodrug of melagatran, was the first oral DTI used in clinical trials from 1999. Its reproducible pharmacokinetic characteristics, rapid onset of action and relatively few interactions with food and other drugs raised hopes that it would allow effective oral anticoagulation without the need for regular international normalized ratio (INR) monitoring. Advanced phase III clinical trials proved ximelagatran to be a potent anticoagulant with ability to prevent venous thromboembolism (VTE) at least as efficiently as injections of the low-molecular-weight heparin (LMWH) enoxaparin followed by administration of warfarin [3]. Ximelagatran was also found to be safe treatment in terms of risk of hemorrhage. However, the randomized, double-blind Thrombin Inhibitor in Venous Thromboembolism Treatment (THRIVE) trial and further studies revealed that treatment with ximelagatran carried substantial risk of hepatotoxicity [4].

On the basis of health concerns ximelagatran did not receive FDA approval and it was subsequently withdrawn by AstraZeneca following the EXTEND study because of fear of liver toxicity [5]. The EXTEND study was terminated due to a case of severe acute liver injury just 3 weeks after completion of the 35-day course of treatment. Even though ximelagatran has been discontinued, it is very important for practitioners to know this information since safety issues of new oral anticoagulants are still a major concern.

Dabigatran etexilate

Dabigatran is a potent nonpeptide DTI but it is not orally active and so its physicochemical characteristics were modified to produce a prodrug, dabigatran etexilate (Figure 5.1). This differs from dabigatran by an ethyl group at the carboxylic acid and a hexyloxycarbonyl side chain at the amidine, and it has strong and long-lasting anticoagulant effects after oral administration [6]. Dabigatran etexilate possesses a number of qualities that make it an attractive anticoagulant. It has rapid absorption (onset of action within 2 hours) and its half-life is approximately 8 hours after single-dose administration and up to 14–17 hours after multiple doses (Table 5.1) [7].

Dabigatran etexilate

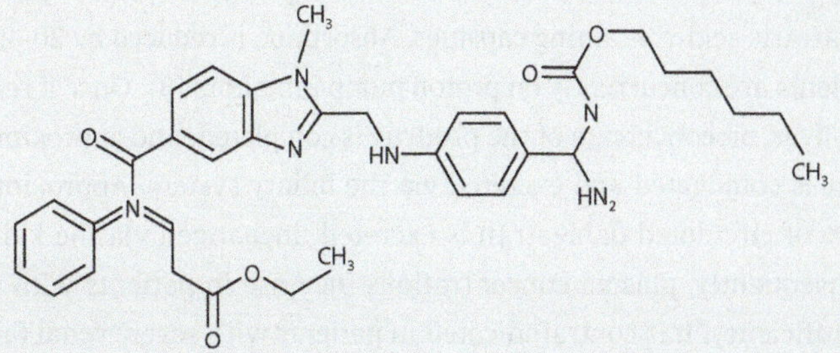

Figure 5.1 Dabigatran etexilate.

Properties of dabigatran etexilate, rivaroxaban, and apixaban

	Dabigatran etexilate	Rivaroxaban	Apixaban
Target	Thrombin	Factor Xa	Factor Xa
Prodrug	Yes	No	No
Bioavailability (%)	6.5	>80	>50
Time to peak level (hours)	2–3	2–4	3
Half-life (hours)	14–17	9	9–14
Renal excretion (%)	80	33 (67% by liver)	25 (~70% in feces)
Dosing	Once or twice daily	Once or twice daily	Twice daily
Drug interactions	Potent CYP3A4 and P-glycoprotein inhibitors	Potent CYP3A4 and P-glycoprotein inhibitors	Potent CYP3A4 and P-glycoprotein inhibitors
Antidote	No	No	No

Table 5.1 Properties of dabigatran etexilate, rivaroxaban, and apixaban.

Dabigatran etexilate is a double prodrug that is converted by esterases into its active metabolite, dabigatran, once it has been absorbed from the gastrointestinal tract. As bioconversion of dabigatran etexilate to dabigatran begins in the gut, the drug enters the portal vein as a combination of prodrug and active compound.

The cytochrome P450 system plays no part in the metabolism of dabigatran etexilate; therefore, the risk of drug interactions is low. Because the bioavailability of dabigatran etexilate is only 6.5%, relatively high doses of the drug must be given to ensure that adequate plasma concentrations are achieved. The absorption of dabigatran etexilate in the stomach and small intestine is dependent on an acid environment. To promote such a microenvironment, dabigatran etexilate is provided in tartaric acid-containing capsules. Absorption is reduced by 20–25% if patients are concurrently on proton pump inhibitors [8]. Once it reaches the liver, bioconversion of the prodrug is completed, and approximately 20% is conjugated and excreted via the biliary system. Approximately 80% of circulated dabigatran is excreted unchanged via the kidneys. Consequently, plasma concentrations increase in patients with renal insufficiency. It is contraindicated in patients with severe renal failure.

It is noteworthy that dabigatran etexilate has no known interactions with food, as well as having a low potential for drug interactions [2]. Accumulated evidence from completed and ongoing trials confirms the hepatic safety of the drug [9].

In March 2008, the European Commission granted marketing authorization for dabigatran etexilate for the prevention of VTE in adults who have undergone total hip replacement (THR) or total knee replacement (TKR). The drug was launched in the UK in April 2008.

Venous thromboembolism prevention in major joint surgery

Clinical evaluation of dabigatran etexilate started in the setting of major joint surgery. In the multicenter, open-label, phase II BISTRO I trial [10], 314 patients undergoing THR were assigned to receive different doses of dabigatran etexilate (12.5, 25, 50, 100, 150, 200, or 300 mg twice daily, or 150 or 300 mg once daily) administered 4–8 hours after surgery for 6–10 days. No major hemorrhages were observed in any group. However, nonmajor multiple-site hemorrhage was observed in two patients with reduced renal clearance treated with the highest dose (300 mg twice daily). The overall incidence of deep vein thrombosis (DVT) was 12.4%, without a consistent relationship between incidence and dose. The lowest dose (12.5 mg twice daily) showed a high rate of proximal DVT (12.5%).

In the subsequent phase II BISTRO II trial [11] the 1973 patients undergoing THR or TKR were randomized to 6–10 days of dabigatran etexilate (50, 150, or 225 mg twice daily, or 300 mg once daily) starting 1–4 hours after surgery, or enoxaparin (40 mg once daily) starting 12 hours prior to surgery. VTE occurred in 28.5, 17.4, 13.1, 16.6, and

24% of patients assigned to dabigatran etexilate 50, 150, 225 mg twice daily, 300 mg once daily, and enoxaparin, respectively. Compared with enoxaparin, VTE was significantly lower in patients receiving 150 or 225 mg twice daily or 300 mg once daily, and major hemorrhage was significantly lower with 50 mg twice daily but elevated with higher doses, nearly achieving statistical significance with the 300 mg once daily dose ($P=0.051$). Together, the BISTRO I and BISTRO II trials showed that dabigatran etexilate might be an effective and safe anticoagulant and served as a basis for dose justification in phase III trials.

The clinical utility of dabigatran etexilate for the prevention of VTE in patients after major joint surgery was confirmed in three large randomized, double-blind, multicenter trials (Table 5.2) [12–15]. The RE-MODEL trial [12] compared dabigatran etexilate (150 mg or 220 mg once daily, starting with a half-dose 1–4 hours after TKR) and enoxaparin (40 mg once daily starting the evening before surgery in 2076 patients). The treatment continued for 6–10 days and patients were followed up for 3 months. The primary efficacy outcome of a composite of total VTE (venographic or symptomatic) and mortality during treatment occurred in 37.7% of patients in the enoxaparin group, 36.4% of the dabigatran etexilate 220 mg group and 40.5% of the 150 mg dabigatran etexilate group. Both dabigatran etexilate doses proved to be noninferior to enoxaparin. The incidence of major hemorrhage also did not differ significantly across the three groups (1.3%, 1.5%, and 1.3%, respectively).

A similar design was used in the RE-NOVATE trial [15] to test potential non-inferiority of dabigatran etexilate for VTE prophylaxis in 3,494 patients undergoing THR, except that the treatment was continued for 28–35 days. The primary efficacy outcome, a composite of total VTE and all-cause mortality during treatment, occurred in 6.7% of individuals in the enoxaparin group, 6.0% of patients in the dabigatran etexilate 220 mg once-daily group, and 8.6% of patients in the 150 mg once-daily group; that is, both the dabigatran etexilate doses were non-inferior to enoxaparin. There was no significant difference in major hemorrhage rates with either dose of dabigatran etexilate compared with enoxaparin. In the phase III RE-NOVATE II trial, the efficacy and safety of oral dabigatran versus subcutaneous enoxaparin was compared for

Efficacy and safety of dabigatran etexilate in major joint surgery

	Duration of treatment	Initiation of dabigatran etexilate	Treatment tested	VTE and all-cause mortality (%)	Major hemorrhage (%)
RE-NOVATE [15] (THA) n=3494	28–35 days	1–4 hours post operation (with half dose)	Dabigatran etexilate 150 mg od	6.7	1.3
			Dabigatran etexilate 220 mg od	8.6	2.0
			Enoxaparin 40 mg od	6.0	1.6
RE-NOVATE II [13] (THA) n=2055	28–35 days	1–4 hours post operation (with half dose)	Dabigatran etexilate 220 mg od	7.7	1.4
			Enoxaparin 40 mg od	8.8	0.9
RE-MODEL [12] (TKA) n=2076	6–10 days	1–4 hours post operation (with half dose)	Dabigatran etexilate	37.7	1.3
			Dabigatran etexilate 220 mg od	40.5	1.5
			Enoxaparin 40 mg od	36.4	1.3
RE-MOBILIZE [14] (TKA) n=1896	12–15 days	6–12 hours post operation	Dabigatran etexilate 150 mg od	25.3	0.6
			Dabigatran etexilate 220 mg od	33.7*	0.6
			Enoxaparin 30 mg bid	31.1*	1.4

Table 5.2 Efficacy and safety of dabigatran etexilate in major joint surgery. Bid, twice daily; od, once daily; THA, total hip arthroplasty; TKA, total knee arthroplasty. *Inferior to enoxaparin. Data from [12–15].

extended thromboprophylaxis in patients undergoing total hip arthroplasty. A total of 2055 patients were randomized. The primary efficacy outcome was a composite of total VTE and death from all causes. The main secondary composite outcome was major VTE plus VTE-related death. The main safety endpoint was major bleeding. The primary efficacy outcome occurred in 7.7% of the dabigatran group versus 8.8% of the enoxaparin group ($P<0.0001$ for the prespecified noninferiority margin).

Major VTE plus VTE-related death occurred in 2.2% of the dabigatran group versus 4.2% of the enoxaparin group. Major bleeding events did not differ between the two arms [13].

No significant differences in the incidences of liver enzyme elevation and acute coronary events were observed during treatment or follow-up in the RE-MODEL or the RE-NOVATE I and II trials.

The successful record of dabigatran etexilate in preceding clinical trials was partly compromised in the double-blind, centrally randomized RE-MOBILIZE trial [14], in which the North American recommended dose for VTE prophylaxis was used for the enoxaparin comparator, (ie, 30 mg twice daily rather than 40 mg once daily). Dabigatran etexilate 220 or 150 mg once daily was compared with enoxaparin 30 mg twice daily after knee arthroplasty surgery. Among 1896 patients, dabigatran etexilate at both doses showed inferior efficacy to enoxaparin, with VTE rates of 31% for 220 mg once daily (P=0.02 versus enoxaparin), 34% for 150 mg once daily (P<0.001 versus enoxaparin), and 25% for enoxaparin. Major hemorrhage was uncommon in all groups: 0.6% for dabigatran 220 mg once daily, 0.6% for dabigatran 150 mg once daily, and 1.4% for enoxaparin (no significant differences). Serious adverse events occurred in 6.9% of dabigatran 220 mg once-daily patients, 6.5% of dabigatran 150 mg once-daily patients, and 5.2% of enoxaparin patients.

An interesting clinical difference between European and North American prophylactic dosing regimens for antithrombotic drugs for perioperative orthopedic patients is that, historically, European dosing regimens administered these drugs before surgery, whereas in North America dosing began postoperatively, sometimes at a higher total daily dosage [16]. Because dabigatran was first investigated in European joint arthroplasty patients, the LMWH control therapy, enoxaparin, was initiated the evening before the day of surgery at the standard dosage of 40 mg once daily in the phase II studies.

Venous thromboembolism treatment
The promising efficacy results for dabigatran in the prevention of thromboembolic disorders prompted the developers to test the drug's utility in VTE treatment (Table 5.3) [10–15,17–20].

Clinical development program for dabigatran etexilate

Clinical condition	Trial	Comparator (n)
VTE prevention in major joint surgery	**Phase II**	
	BISTRO I [10]	No comparator (314)
	BISTRO II [11]	Enoxaparin (1973)
	Phase III	
	RE-MODEL [12]	Enoxaparin (2076)
	RE-NOVATE [15]	Enoxaparin (3494)
	RE-MOBILIZE [14]	Enoxaparin (1896)
	RE-NOVATE II [13]	Enoxaparin (1920)
VTE treatment	**Phase III**	
	RE-COVER [17]	Parenteral anticoagulant/ warfarin (2564)
	NCT00680186	Parenteral anticoagulant/ warfarin (2554)
	RE-SONATE (NCT00558259)	Placebo (1547)
	RE-MEDY (NCT00329238)	Warfarin (2500)
Stroke prevention in atrial fibrillation	**Phase II**	
	PETRO [18]	Aspirin or warfarin (502)
	Phase III	
	RE-LY [19]	Warfarin (18,000)
	RELY-ABLE (NCT00808067)	Placebo (6200)
Acute coronary syndrome	RE-DEEM [20]	Placebo (1878)
Percutaneous coronary intervention	NCT00818753	Heparin (50)

Table 5.3 Clinical development program for dabigatran etexilate. VTE, venous thromboembolism. Data from [10–15,17–20] and www.clinicaltrials.gov for ongoing clinical trial information.

The RE-COVER study was a randomized, double-blind, noninferiority trial involving 1274 patients with acute VTE who were initially given parenteral anticoagulation therapy for a median of 9 days [17]. The RE-COVER population was assigned to dabigatran, administered at a dose of 150 mg twice daily, or dose-adjusted warfarin. The primary outcome was the 6-month incidence of recurrent VTE and related deaths. Safety endpoints included bleeding events, acute coronary syndromes (ACSs), other adverse events, and results of liver-function tests. The RE-COVER investigators concluded that for the treatment of acute VTE, a fixed dose of dabigatran is as effective as warfarin (primary outcome rate 2.4%

versus 2.1%, respectively; $P<0.001$ for the prespecified noninferiority margin) and has a safety profile that is similar to that of warfarin [17].

In a separate phase III randomized multicenter trial, RE-SONATE, the efficacy of prolonged (additional 12 months) administration of dabigatran etexilate in 1547 patients with VTE was compared with placebo. In RE-SONATE, extended treatment with dabigatran was associated with a 92% relative risk reduction for recurrent VTE and a low risk for major bleeding [21]. Additionally, the RE-MEDY trial aimed to evaluate the comparative safety and efficacy of dabigatran etexilate and warfarin for the long-term treatment and secondary prevention of symptomatic VTE in patients who have already been successfully treated with a standard anticoagulant approach for 3–6 months for confirmed acute symptomatic VTE. In RE-MEDY, dabigatran demonstrated noninferiority to warfarin for the outcome of recurrent VTE, with fewer bleeds, but there were more acute coronary syndrome events in the dabigatran group than in those taking warfarin [22].

Stroke prevention in atrial fibrillation

The clinical safety of dabigatran etexilate (with or without aspirin) in patients with atrial fibrillation (AF) was first assessed in the phase II dose-range Prevention of Embolic and ThROmbotic Events in Patients with Persistent Atrial Fibrillation (PETRO) trial [18]. In this trial, 502 patients with AF were randomized to receive dabigatran etexilate 50, 150, or 300 mg twice daily alone or combined with 81 mg or 325 mg of aspirin or warfarin once daily for 12 weeks. Major hemorrhage was limited to the group treated with 300 mg dabigatran plus aspirin (4 of 64), and the incidence was significant versus 300 mg dabigatran alone (0 of 105, $P<0.02$). Total hemorrhage events were more frequent in the 300 mg (23%) and 150 mg (18%) dabigatran groups compared with the 50 mg groups (7%; $P=0.0002$ and $P=0.01$, respectively). The study demonstrated that major hemorrhages were limited to patients treated with dabigatran 300 mg plus aspirin, and thromboembolic episodes were limited to the 50 mg dabigatran groups. On the basis of the PETRO study, 150 mg and 220 mg doses were chosen for further development in phase III studies of stroke prevention in AF.

The Randomized Evaluation of Long term anticoagulant therapy (RE-LY) with dabigatran etexilate trial compared the efficacy and safety of two doses of dabigatran etexilate with warfarin in over 18,000 patients with AF with an average age of 71 years. The primary outcome measure was the incidence of stroke (including hemorrhagic) or systemic embolism at the median 2-year follow-up period. Treatment with the higher, 150 mg twice daily dose significantly reduced the rate of stroke and systemic embolism (with a relative risk of 0.66, $P<0.001$; the rate of hemorrhagic stroke was 0.38% per year in the warfarin group versus 0.10% per year with dabigatran, $P<0.001$), with a similar overall risk to warfarin for major bleeding [19]. The lower, 110 mg twice daily dose resulted in a similar risk for stroke as warfarin but with a significantly reduced major bleeding event rate (20% relative risk reduction, 3.36% per year in the warfarin group versus 2.71% per year with dabigatran, $P=0.003$). The rate of hemorrhagic stroke was 0.38% per year in the warfarin group, as compared with 0.12% per year with 110 mg dabigatran ($P<0.001$) and 0.10% per year with 150 mg of dabigatran ($P<0.001$). Annual mortality rate was 4.13% in the warfarin group, 3.75% with 110 mg of dabigatran and 3.64% with 150 mg of dabigatran (borderline significance, $P=0.051$) [19] (Figure 5.2). The long-term extension study, RELY-ABLE, is investigating the safety of more prolonged treatment with dabigatran etexilate in those who completed the RE-LY trial, with a recruitment target of 6200 patients.

In view of the results of the RE-LY trial, dabigatran has been included in the latest European guidelines for management of AF as an alternative to vitamin K antagonists (VKAs) for primary or secondary prevention of stroke in patients with AF. The US Food and Drug Administration (FDA) approved in October 2010 the 150 mg twice-daily dosage, which should be reduced to 75 mg twice daily in selected cases (eg, creatinine clearance 15–30 ml/minute). Dabigatran was recently licensed by the European Medicines Agency (EMA) at two dosages (110 mg and 150 mg twice daily), depending on the balance between thromboembolic and bleeding risk factors.

Other directions

The potential application of DTIs is not limited in conditions related to venous thrombosis, and dabigatran etexilate has also been tested in

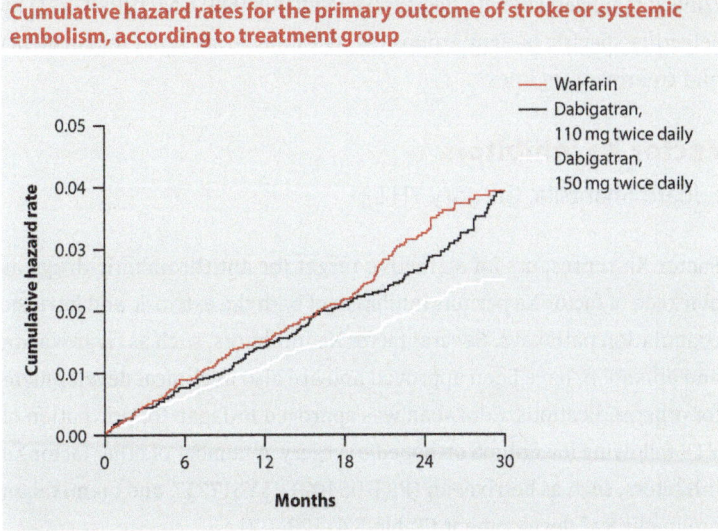

Cumulative hazard rates for the primary outcome of stroke or systemic embolism, according to treatment group

Figure 5.2 Cumulative hazard rates for the primary outcome of stroke or systemic embolism, according to treatment group. Reproduced with permission from Connolly et al [19].

phase II trials in clinical settings of arterial thrombosis. In a randomized, open-label study of dabigatran etexilate in elective percutaneous coronary intervention (NCT00818753) two doses of dabigatran etexilate (110 mg and 150 mg twice daily) were compared with heparin (both in addition to a standard dual antiplatelet regimen) in 50 patients undergoing elective percutaneous coronary intervention; the results of this study have not been published as yet. RE-DEEM (Dose-Finding Study for Dabigatran Etexilate in Patients With Acute Coronary Syndrome), a larger (n=1878) placebo-controlled trial, evaluated the safety and potential of efficacy of four different dabigatran doses administered twice daily for 6 months in addition to dual antiplatelet treatment in patients with ACS at high risk of cardiovascular complications [20]. In the RE-DEEM study dabigatran, in addition to dual antiplatelet therapy, was associated with a dose-dependent increase in bleeding events compared with placebo and significantly reduced coagulation activity in patients with a recent myocardial infarction [20].

Additionally, the safety and tolerability of dabigatran etexilate has been evaluated in adolescent patients with VTE (phase II trial NCT00844415), and a number of observational cohort studies aimed to further optimize clinical management with dabigatran (NCT00846807, NCT00847301) by selecting specific patient groups (eg, with moderate renal impairment) and treatment regimes.

Factor Xa inhibitors
Eduard Shantsila, Gregory YH Lip

Factor Xa represents an attractive target for antithrombotic drugs as blockade of factor Xa permits inhibition of both the extrinsic and intrinsic coagulation pathways. Several factor Xa inhibitors, such as rivaroxaban and apixaban, have been approved and are also in clinical development for other indications. Edoxaban was approved in Japan for prevention of VTE following lower-limb orthopedic surgery. A number of other factor Xa inhibitors, such as betrixaban (PRT-054021), LY517717, and otamixaban are in clinical development (Table 5.4) [23–27].

Rivaroxaban
Rivaroxaban (Figure 5.3) is a novel factor Xa inhibitor that exhibits predictable pharmacokinetics, with high oral bioavailability, rapid onset

Clinical development of the emerging factor Xa inhibitors			
Clinical condition	**Phase**	**Trial title**	**Comparator (n)**
Betrixaban (PRT054021)			
VTE prevention in major joint surgery	II	Factor Xa Inhibitor, PRT054021, Against Enoxaparin for the Prevention of Venous Thromboembolic Events (EXPERT) [23]	Enoxaparin (200)
Stroke prevention in atrial fibrillation	II	Study of the Safety, Tolerability and Pilot Efficacy of Oral Factor Xa Inhibitor Betrixaban Compared to Warfarin (EXPLORE-Xa) [24]	Warfarin (500)
Edoxaban (DU-176b)			
VTE prevention in major joint surgery	II	A Study of DU-176b in Preventing Blood Clots After Hip Replacement Surgery [25]	Not specified in trial (402)
	II	Study of the Efficacy and Safety of DU-176b in Preventing Blood Clots in Patients Undergoing Total Hip Replacement (NCT 00398216)	Dalteparin (950)

Table 5.4 Clinical development of the emerging factor Xa inhibitors (continue opposite).

Clinical development of the emerging factor Xa inhibitors (continued)

Clinical condition	Phase	Trial title	Comparator (n)
Stroke prevention in atrial fibrillation	II	A Study to Assess the Safety of a Potential New Drug in Comparison to the Standard Practice of Dosing With Warfarin for Non-Valvular Atrial Fibrillation (NCT00504556)	Warfarin (2000)
	II	DU-176b Phase 2 Dose Finding Study in Subjects With Non-Valvular Atrial Fibrillation (NCT00806624)	Warfarin (235)
	II	Late Phase 2 Study of DU-176b in Patients With Non-Valvular Atrial Fibrillation (NCT00829933)	Warfarin (536)
VTE prevention in major joint surgery	III	STARS E-3 trial: a study of edoxaban for the prevention of venous thromboembolism in patients after total knee arthroplasty (NCT01181102)	Enoxaparin (716)
	III	STARS J-V trial: a study of edoxaban for the prevention of venous thromboembolism in patients after total hip arthroplasty (NCT01181167)	Enoxaparin (610)
VTE treatment	III	HOKUSAI VTE trial: a study of edoxaban for the treatment and prevention of recurrent VTE in patients with DVT and/or PE (NCT00986154)	Enoxaparin/ warfarin (8250)
Stroke/systemic embolic events	III	Global Study to Assess the Safety and Effectiveness of Edoxaban (DU-176b) vs Standard Practice of Dosing With Warfarin in Patients With Atrial Fibrillation (EngageAFTIMI48)	Warfarin (16,500)
LY517717			
VTE prevention in major joint surgery	II	New Oral Anticoagulant Therapy for the Prevention of Blood Clots Following Hip or Knee Replacement Surgery [26]	Enoxaparin (511)
Otamixaban (XRP0673)			
Percutaneous coronary intervention	II	The SEPIA-PCI Trial: Otamixaban in Comparison to Heparin in Subjects Undergoing Non-Urgent Percutaneous Coronary Intervention (NCT00133731)	Unfractionated heparin (947)
Non-ST elevation acute coronary syndrome	II	Study of Otamixaban Versus Unfractionated Heparin (UFH) and Eptifibatide in Non-ST Elevation Acute Coronary Syndrome (SEPIA-ACS1) [27]	Unfractionated heparin, eptifibatide (3240)

Table 5.4 Clinical development of the emerging factor Xa inhibitors (continued). VTE, venous thromboembolism. Data from [23–27] and www.clinicaltrials.gov for ongoing trial information.

Rivaroxaban

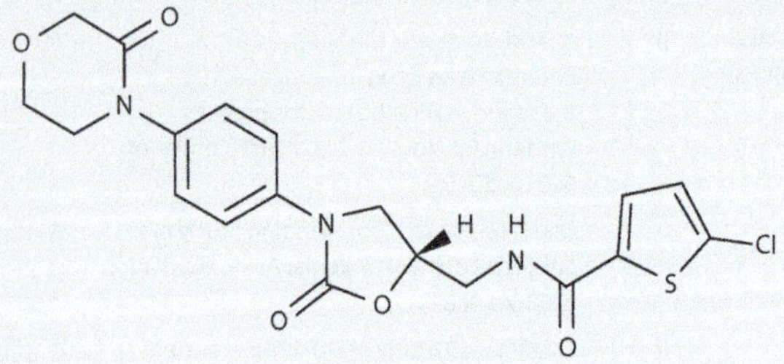

Figure 5.3 Rivaroxaban.

of action (achieves maximum plasma concentration in 1.5–2.0 hours), and no known food interactions [28] (see Table 5.3). The drug has a dual mode of elimination: two-thirds of it is metabolized by the liver (mostly via CYP3A4 and CYP2J2), with no major or active circulating metabolites identified, and one-third is excreted unchanged by the kidneys. Elimination of rivaroxaban from plasma occurs with a terminal half-life of 5–9 hours in young individuals, and with a terminal half-life of 12–13 hours in subjects aged >75 years [29]. Available data indicate that body weight, age, and gender do not have a clinically relevant effect on the pharmacokinetics and pharmacodynamics of rivaroxaban, and it thus can be administered in fixed doses without coagulation monitoring. Rivaroxaban has minimal drug interactions (eg, with naproxen, acetylsalicylic acid, clopidogrel, or digoxin) [28] and its predictable pharmacokinetics and pharmacodynamics allow use of rivaroxaban without regular laboratory monitoring. Although no specific antidote is known for rivaroxaban, preclinical data suggested that recombinant factor VIIa and activated prothrombin complex concentrate may reverse the effects of high-dose rivaroxaban [30–32].

Venous thromboembolism prevention

Four completed phase II efficacy and safety studies of rivaroxaban for the prevention of VTE in patients undergoing elective THR and TKR (n=2907 patients) have demonstrated comparable efficacy and safety of rivaroxaban and conventional management with subcutaneous enoxaparin [33–36].

Efficacy was assessed as a composite of any DVT (proximal or distal), nonfatal objectively confirmed PE and all-cause mortality; safety was judged on the basis of major hemorrhage incidence. A pooled analysis of two of these studies confirmed non-inferiority of rivaroxaban in patients undergoing elective THR or TKR, with no significant dose–response relationship for efficacy but with a significant dose-related increase for the primary safety endpoint ($P<0.001$), a total daily dose of 5–20 mg being the optimal dose range (Figure 5.4) [33,37].

Consequently, a fixed dose of rivaroxaban 10 mg once daily was selected to be used in the phase III RECORD (REgulation of Coagulation in ORthopedic surgery to prevent DVT and PE) program (Table 5.5) [38–41]. The RECORD program included four large trials that recruited more than 12,500 patients undergoing elective THR or TKR. All RECORD

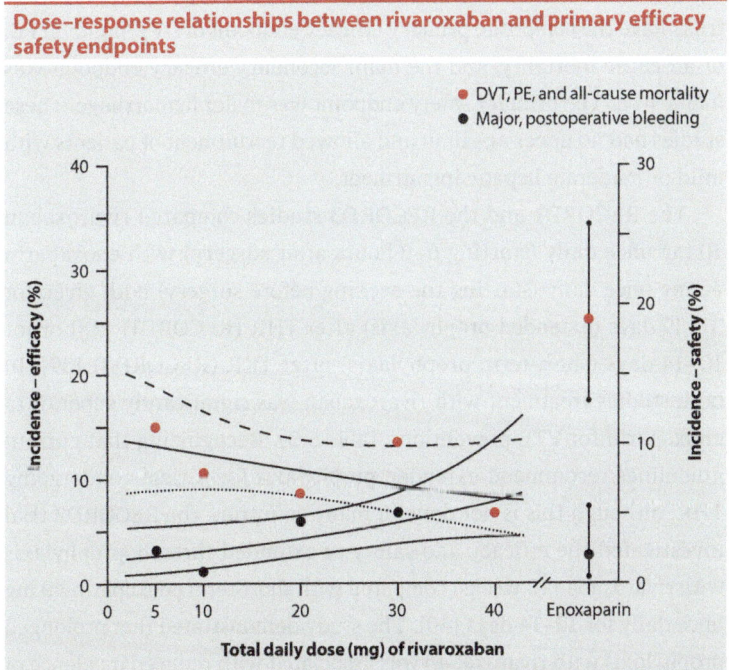

Dose–response relationships between rivaroxaban and primary efficacy safety endpoints

- ● DVT, PE, and all-cause mortality
- ● Major, postoperative bleeding

Figure 5.4 Dose–response relationships between rivaroxaban and primary efficacy safety endpoints. Results for the prevention of venous thromboembolism after major orthopedic surgery. DVT, deep vein thrombosis; PE, pulmonary embolism. Reproduced with permission from Eriksson et al [33].

Incidence of venous thromboembolism and hemorrhage in the RECORD program

Trial	Regimen (once daily)	Duration of treatment	Total VTE (%)	P
RECORD1 (THR) n=4541 [38]	Rivaroxaban 10 mg	5 weeks	1.1	<0.001
	Enoxaparin 40 mg	5 weeks	3.7	
RECORD2 (THR) n=2509 [40]	Rivaroxaban 10 mg	10–14 days	2.0	<0.0001
	Enoxaparin 40 mg	5 weeks	9.3	
RECORD3 (TKR) n=2531 [39]	Rivaroxaban 10 mg	10–14 days	9.6	<0.001
	Enoxaparin 40 mg	10–14 days	18.9	
RECORD4 (TKR) n=3148 [41]	Rivaroxaban 10 mg	10–14 days	6.9	0.012
	Enoxaparin 40 mg	10–14 days	10.1	

Table 5.5 Incidence of venous thromboembolism and hemorrhage in the RECORD program. NA, not available; THR, total hip replacement; TKR, total knee replacement; VTE, venous thromboembolism. Data from [38–41].

trials have the composite primary efficacy endpoint of DVT, nonfatal PE, or all-cause mortality, and the main secondary efficacy endpoint was major VTE. The primary safety endpoint was major hemorrhage. These studies had no upper age limit and allowed recruitment of patients with mild or moderate hepatic impairment.

The RECORD1 and the RECORD3 studies compared rivaroxaban 10 mg once daily (starting 6–8 hours after surgery) with enoxaparin 40 mg once daily (starting the evening before surgery) both given for 31–39 days (extended prophylaxis) after THR (RECORD1) [38] or for 10–14 days (short-term prophylaxis) after TKR (RECORD3) [39]. In both studies treatment with rivaroxaban was significantly superior to enoxaparin for VTE prevention (Table 5.5). Recognizing that current guidelines recommend extended prophylaxis for patients undergoing THR, although this is not done in many countries, the RECORD2 trial investigated the efficacy and safety of extended thromboprophylaxis with rivaroxaban (5 weeks) compared with short-term enoxaparin 40 mg once daily for 10–14 days [40]. The study demonstrated that prolonged prophylaxis with rivaroxaban was associated with reduced incidence of VTE, including symptomatic events, after THR. Of note, despite administration of rivaroxaban for 3 weeks longer than enoxaparin, the rate of major hemorrhage at 5 weeks was low and similar in both groups.

Major VTE		Symptomatic VTE		Major hemorrhage	Clinically relevant nonmajor hemorrhage
(%)	P	(%)	P	(%)	
0.2	<0.001	0.3	0.22	0.3	2.9
2.0		0.5		0.1	2.4
0.6	<0.0001	0.2	0.004	<0.1	3.3
5.1		1.2		<0.1	2.7
1.0	0.01	0.7	0.005	0.6	2.7
2.6		2.0		0.5	2.3
1.2	0.124	0.7	0.187	0.7	NA
2.0		1.2		0.3	NA

In the RECORD4 trial rivaroxaban 10 mg was significantly more effective than the North American regimen of enoxaparin 30 mg twice daily (10–14 days) for the prevention of VTE in patients undergoing TKR, with similar rates of major hemorrhage for both treatments and no serious liver toxicity with rivaroxaban [41]. Thus, the superiority of rivaroxaban over enoxaparin for VTE prevention was demonstrated in all four studies, with a good safety profile. As a result, in 2008 rivaroxaban received approval in the European Union and in Canada for the prevention of VTE in patients undergoing elective THR or TKR surgery. In July 2011, the FDA approved rivaroxaban for prophylaxis of DVT in adults undergoing hip and knee replacement surgery.

The utility of rivaroxaban (10 mg once daily for up to 5 weeks) for VTE prevention in hospitalized medically ill patients is currently being assessed in a phase III MAGELLAN study, with short-term enoxaparin as the comparator [42].

Treatment of venous thromboembolism

The initial phase IIb ODIXa-DVT [43] and EINSTEIN-DVT [44] studies (Table 5.6) assessed the clinical efficacy and safety of rivaroxaban for the treatment of VTE in patients with acute, symptomatic, proximal DVT without symptomatic PE. The treatment was administered for

Clinical efficacy and safety of rivaroxaban for the treatment of venous thromboembolism

ODIXa-DVT study

	Rivaroxaban				Enoxaparin + VKA
	10 mg bid (n=100)	20 mg bid (n=98)	30 mg bid (n=109)	40 mg bid (n=112)	(n=109)
Improvement in thrombus burden without recurrent VTE at 3 weeks (%)	53.0	59.2	56.9	43.8	45.9
Recurrent DVT, PE, and VTE-related death at 3 months, n (%)	2 (1.9)	2 (2.0)	2 (1.8)	3 (2.6)	1 (0.9)
Major hemorrhage, n (%)	2 (1.7)	2 (1.7)	4 (3.3)	2 (1.7)	0

EINSTEIN-DVT study

	Rivaroxaban			LMWH/heparin + VKA
	20 mg od (n=115)	30 mg od (n=112)	40 mg od (n=121)	(n=101)
Recurrent VTE and thrombus deterioration at 3 months, n (%)	7 (6.1)	6 (5.4)	8 (6.6)	10 (9.9)
Major hemorrhage, n (%)	1 (0.7)	2 (1.5)	0 (0.0)	2 (1.5)

Table 5.6 Clinical efficacy and safety of rivaroxaban for the treatment of venous thromboembolism. DVT, deep vein thrombosis; LMWH, low-molecular-weight heparin; od, once daily; PE, pulmonary embolism; VKA, vitamin K antagonist; VTE, venous thromboembolism. Data from Agnelli et al [43] and Buller et al [44].

3 months, with open-label standard therapy (LMWH/heparin following VKA) as comparator.

In the ODIXa-DVT study, rivaroxaban doses 10, 20, or 30 mg twice daily, or 40 mg once daily, were tested [43]. The primary efficacy endpoint of reduced thrombus burden on day 21 (assessed by quantitative compression ultrasonography) without recurrent VTE or VTE-related death was reported in 43.8–59.2% of patients receiving rivaroxaban and in 45.9% of patients receiving standard therapy. The incidence of the primary safety endpoint (major hemorrhage) was 1.7–3.3% in the rivaroxaban groups; there were no events in the standard therapy group.

In the EINSTEIN-DVT study [44], therapy with rivaroxaban 20–40 mg once daily was associated with an incidence of 5.4–6.6% for the primary endpoint (the composite of symptomatic, recurrent VTE, and deterioration of thrombotic burden, as assessed by compression ultrasound and perfusion lung scan) compared with 9.9% in the standard therapy group. The primary safety endpoint (any clinically relevant hemorrhage) developed in 2.9–7.5% of patients receiving rivaroxaban and 8.8% of those on the standard therapy, with no evidence of compromised liver function in those receiving rivaroxaban.

Of note, the phase II studies revealed that the twice-daily rivaroxaban regimen was more effective for thrombus regression at 3 weeks, whereas the once- and twice-daily regimens showed similar effectiveness at 3-month follow-up [43]. Accordingly, an initial intensified twice-daily regimen (rivaroxaban 15 mg twice daily for 3 weeks) followed by long-term 20 mg once-daily dosing was chosen for investigation in the phase III EINSTEIN studies: EINSTEIN-DVT, EINSTEIN-PE, and EINSTEIN-EXTENSION [44–47].

EINSTEIN-DVT was an open-label, randomized, event-driven, non-inferiority study that compared oral rivaroxaban (15 mg twice daily for 3 weeks, followed by 20 mg once daily) against subcutaneous enoxaparin followed by a VKA for 3, 6, or 12 months in patients with acute, symptomatic DVT [44]. In parallel, EINSTEIN-EXTENSION was a double-blind, randomized, event-driven superiority study that compared rivaroxaban alone (20 mg once daily) with placebo for an additional 6 or 12 months in patients who had completed 6 to 12 months of treatment for VTE [46]. The primary efficacy outcome for both studies was recurrent VTE. The principal safety outcome for EINSTEIN-DVT was major bleeding or clinically relevant nonmajor bleeding in the initial-treatment study and major bleeding in the continued-treatment study. The study recruited 3449 patients: 1731 in the rivaroxaban arm and 1718 in the conventional management arm [47]. Rivaroxaban was noninferior with respect to the primary efficacy outcome while the principal safety outcome occurred in 8.1% of the patients in each group. In the extended-treatment study, which included 602 patients in the rivaroxaban group and 594 in the placebo group, rivaroxaban had superior efficacy. Four patients in the rivaroxaban group had nonfatal major bleeding (0.7%), versus none in the placebo group ($P=0.11$) [47].

In December 2011 rivaroxaban received approval by the European Commission for treatment of DVT and prevention of recurrent DVT and pulmonary embolism following an acute DVT in adults. Phase III clinical development programs for rivaroxaban are outlined in Table 5.7 [42,44–46,48–50].

In the recently published randomized, open-label, event-driven, noninferiority EINSTEIN-PE trial 4832 subjects with acute symptomatic PE with or without DVT were assigned to either rivaroxaban (15 mg twice daily for 3 weeks, followed by 20 mg once daily) or to standard therapy with enoxaparin followed by dose-adjusted VKA for 3, 6, or 12 months [45]. The trial demonstrated that rivaroxaban was noninferior to standard therapy for the primary efficacy outcome symptomatic recurrent VTE (2.1% versus 1.8%, respectively, $P=0.003$ for noninferiority margin). Also, 10.3% of patients treated with rivaroxaban developed the principal safety outcome of major or clinically relevant nonmajor bleeding versus 11.4% in those on standard care ($P=0.23$), thus suggesting that fixed-dose rivaroxaban can be an effective and safe therapeutic option in PE.

Phase III clinical development programs for rivaroxaban		
Clinical condition	**Trial**	**Comparator**
VTE prevention in medically ill patients	MAGELLAN [42]	Standard enoxaparin therapy
Stroke prevention in atrial fibrillation	ROCKET AF [48]	Standard warfarin therapy
	J-ROCKET [50]	
Secondary prevention of cardiovascular events in acute coronary syndrome	ATLAS ACS 2–TIMI 51 [49]	Placebo, in addition to standard therapy
VTE treatment	EINSTEIN-DVT [44]	Vitamin K antagonists
	EINSTEIN-PE [45]	
	EINSTEIN-EXTENSION [46]	

Table 5.7 **Phase III clinical development programs for rivaroxaban.** VTE, venous thromboembolism. Data from [42,44–46,48–50] and www.clinicaltrials.gov for ongoing trial information.

Stroke prevention in atrial fibrillation

In terms of numbers of patients, stroke prevention in AF is potentially the largest indication that may benefit from the novel oral anticoagulants. The rising incidence of AF in a progressively aging population suggests that millions of people may eventually require life-long anticoagulant therapy to prevent severely disabling complications. The ROCKET AF study investigated the effectiveness and safety of rivaroxaban 20 mg once daily (15 mg once daily in those with moderate kidney impairment) versus warfarin for the prevention of stroke or systemic embolism in 14,264 patients with nonvalvular AF who were at an increased risk for stroke [48]. Rivaroxaban was noninferior to warfarin for the prevention of stroke or systemic embolism (hazard ratio in the rivaroxaban group, 0.79; 95% confidence interval [CI], 0.66-0.96; P<0.001 for noninferiority). Moreover, there was no significant between-group difference in the risk of major bleeding, although intracranial and fatal bleeding occurred less frequently in the rivaroxaban group [48]. In the J-ROCKET AF study conducted in Japan, a lower dose of rivaroxaban (15 mg once daily; 5 mg once daily for patients with moderate renal impairment) was shown to be non-inferior to warfarin for the prevention of stroke or systemic embolism [50].

In November 2011, in view of the results of the ROCKET AF study, rivaroxaban was approved by the FDA for the prevention of stroke and systemic embolism in patients with nonvalvular AF, at a dose of 20 mg (or 15 mg if creatinine clearance 15–50 ml/min) once daily. In December 2011, rivaroxaban was approved by the European Commission for prevention of stroke and systemic embolism in adult patients with nonvalvular AF with one or more risk factors.

Acute coronary syndromes

Preclinical data indicated the possible effectiveness of rivaroxaban and other factor Xa inhibitors and DTIs in clinical settings of arterial thrombosis [51]. In the phase IIb ATLAS ACS-TIMI 46 (Anti-Xa Therapy to Lower cardiovascular events in Addition to aspirin with/without thienopyridine therapy in Subjects with Acute Coronary Syndrome) study, 3491 patients with recent ACS were randomized to escalating total daily doses of rivaroxaban, ranging from 5 mg up to 20 mg (once or twice daily), or placebo, in addition to the standard antiplatelet therapy of aspirin or aspirin plus a thienopyridine (eg, clopidogrel) for secondary prevention of cardiovascular events [52]. Patients on the rivaroxaban regimens had higher rates of hemorrhage than those on placebo, and the risk increased in a dose-dependent manner; however, no study arm was stopped due to increased hemorrhage. A strong trend towards reduction in cardiovascular events was observed with rivaroxaban, which reduced the main secondary efficacy endpoint of death, myocardial infarction, or stroke compared with placebo ($P=0.0270$). Two doses of rivaroxaban were tested in the phase III ATLAS ACS 2–TIMI 51 study [49]. The study assigned 15,526 patients with a recent ACS to receive twice-daily doses of either 2.5 mg or 5 mg of rivaroxaban or placebo for a mean of 13 months and up to 31 months. The primary efficacy endpoint was a composite of death from cardiovascular causes, myocardial infarction, or stroke. The investigators concluded that in patients with a recent ACS, rivaroxaban reduced the risk of the composite endpoint (8.9% versus 10.7%, $P=0.008$) and increased the risk of major bleeding (2.1% versus 0.6%, $P<0.001$) and intracranial hemorrhage (0.6% versus 0.2%, $P=0.009$) but not the risk of fatal bleeding [49].

Apixaban

Apixaban is another potent, highly selective, and reversible inhibitor of factor Xa and is active against both free enzyme and factor Xa bound within the prothrombinase complex (Figure 5.5). The bioavailability of apixaban after oral absorption is over 50% [53]. Peak plasma levels of apixaban are observed 3 hours after administration and plasma concentrations reach the steady state by day 3. The half-life of apixaban is between 8 and 15 hours, which allows twice-daily administration of the drug. The primary elimination route is fecal, with only about 25% eliminated via the kidney. Apixaban has little effect on the prothrombin time at therapeutic concentrations, but plasma levels can be assessed using a factor Xa inhibition assay. The clinical development program of apixaban is summarized in Table 5.8 [54–61].

Apixaban

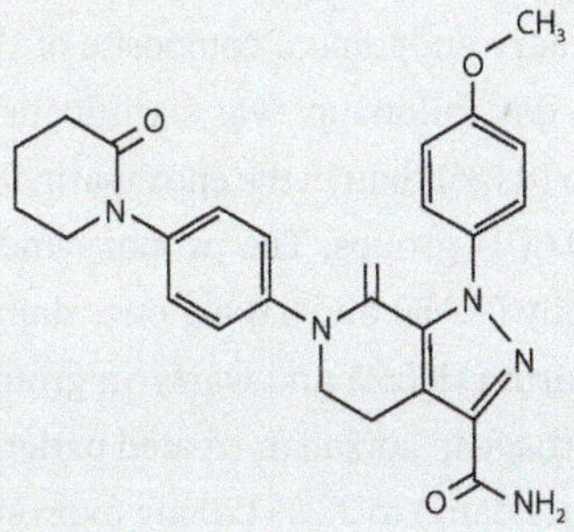

Figure 5.5 Apixaban.

Clinical development of apixaban

Clinical condition	Trial	Comparator
Total knee replacement	ADVANCE-1 [54]	Enoxaparin
	ADVANCE-2 [55]	Enoxaparin
Total hip replacement	ADVANCE-3 [56]	Enoxaparin
Stroke prevention in atrial fibrillation	AVERROES [58]	Aspirin
	ARISTOTLE [57]	Warfarin
Thromboprophylaxis in cancer	ADVOCATE (NCT00320255)	Placebo
Thromboprophylaxis in heart failure, acute respiratory failure or infection (without septic shock), or acute rheumatic disorder or inflammatory bowel disease	ADOPT [59]	Enoxaparin
VTE treatment	AMPLIFY (NCT00643201)	Enoxaparin/warfarin
	AMPLIFY-EXT (NCT00633893)	Placebo
Acute coronary syndrome	Phase II APPRAISE-1 [60]	Placebo
Acute coronary syndrome	Phase III APPRAISE-2 [61]	Placebo

Table 5.8 Clinical development of apixaban. VTE, venous thromboembolism. Data from [54–61] and www.clinicaltrials.gov for information from ongoing trials.

Venous thromboembolism prevention in major joint surgery

In a randomized phase II dose-response clinical trial in 1238 patients undergoing TKR, apixaban 5, 10, or 20 mg/day (administered as once or twice daily doses) was compared with enoxaparin (30 mg twice daily) and open-label warfarin [62]. Apixaban and enoxaparin were started 12–24 hours after surgery; the warfarin dose was titrated from the evening of the day of surgery. After 10–14 days of the treatment, bilateral venography was performed and patients were further treated at the attending physician's discretion. The primary endpoint, a composite of VTE events plus all-cause mortality at 42-day follow-up, was significantly lower in the compound apixaban group (8.6%) than in the enoxaparin (15.6%, $P<0.02$) or warfarin (26.6%, $P<0.001$) groups. The primary endpoint rates for 2.5 mg apixaban twice daily (9.9%) and 5.0 mg once daily (11.3%) were lower than in the enoxaparin (15.6%) and warfarin group (26.6%). The incidence of major hemorrhage in apixaban-treated patients was low and ranged from 0 (2.5 mg twice daily) to 3.3% (20 mg four times daily), with comparable results for once- and twice-daily administration. No major hemorrhage was observed in the enoxaparin and warfarin groups [62].

The clinical utility of apixaban for VTE prevention after major joint surgery was investigated in the phase III ADVANCE program (Table 5.8). In two multicenter, randomized, double-blind, active-controlled clinical trials (ADVANCE-1 and ADVANCE-2), the safety and efficacy of oral apixaban (2.5 mg twice daily) versus enoxaparin (30 mg twice daily in ADVANCE-1 and 40 mg once daily in ADVANCE-2) for preventing DVT and PE after TKR was evaluated in 3195 patients in ADVANCE-1 and 3057 patients in ADVANCE-2 [54,55]. The duration of treatment was 12 days and the primary outcome of both studies was defined as a combination of asymptomatic and symptomatic DVT, nonfatal PE and all-cause mortality. In ADVANCE-1, apixaban did not meet the prespecified statistical criteria for noninferiority versus enoxaparin, but its use was associated with lower rates of clinically relevant bleeding and it had a similar adverse-event profile [54]. In ADVANCE-2, apixaban 2.5 mg twice daily, starting the morning after TKR, offered a more effective orally administered alternative to 40 mg per day enoxaparin (relative risk 0.62 [95% CI 0.51–0.74]; $P<0.0001$), without increased bleeding rates [55].

Similarly, in the ADVANCE-3 trial, the efficacy and safety of 5-week administration of apixaban (2.5 mg twice daily) in comparison with enoxaparin in the prevention of DVT and PE was assessed in 5407 patients after THR. Patients were randomized to receive apixaban plus placebo or enoxaparin plus placebo for 5 weeks. The primary outcome was again a combination of asymptomatic and symptomatic DVT, nonfatal PE, and all-cause mortality. The ADVANCE-3 investigators concluded that, among patients undergoing hip replacement, apixaban was associated with lower rates of VTE without increased bleeding compared to subcutaneous enoxaparin (relative risk with apixaban, 0.36; 95% confidence interval [CI], 0.22 to 0.54; $P<0.001$ for both noninferiority and superiority) [56]. Apixaban received approval in the European Union for the prevention of VTE in patients undergoing elective THR or TKR surgery in May 2011.

Stroke prevention in atrial fibrillation

Two phase III clinical trials assessed apixaban for stroke prevention in patients with AF. In the first, the AVERROES study, the effectiveness of oral apixaban (5.0 mg twice daily; or 2.5 mg in selected patients) was compared with aspirin (81–324 mg once daily) for 36 months in the prevention of stroke or systemic embolism in 5599 patients with permanent or persistent AF who had at least one additional risk factor for stroke but could not be treated with VKA [58]. The data and safety monitoring board recommended early termination of the study because of a clear benefit in favor of apixaban. Apixaban compared to aspirin reduced the risk of stroke or systemic embolism (1.6% versus 3.7% per year, respectively, $P<0.001$) without significantly increasing the risk of major bleeding or intracranial hemorrhage [58].

The second phase III trial, the ARISTOTLE study, investigated whether apixaban (5 mg twice daily) was as effective as warfarin in preventing stroke and systemic embolism in 18,201 patients with AF who had at least one additional risk factor for stroke [57]. The primary efficacy endpoint was the composite outcome of stroke or systemic embolism. In ARISTOTLE, apixaban reduced the risk of stroke or systemic embolism by 21% compared to warfarin. The reduction was significant ($P<0.01$) and supported the superiority of apixaban over warfarin for the primary outcome of preventing stroke or systemic embolism. Apixaban also reduced all-cause mortality by 11% and major bleeding by 31% [57]. Apixaban has become the first new oral anticoagulant superior to warfarin in reducing stroke or systemic embolism, all-cause mortality, and major bleeding in patients with AF. Apixaban received approval by the European Commission for the prevention of stroke and systemic embolism in patients with non-valvular AF in November 2012 and by the FDA in December 2012.

Thromboprophylaxis in other clinical settings

Apixaban is being tested in several additional settings, which may expand the use of oral anticoagulation beyond currently established indications. The phase II randomized ADVOCATE study has been designed to determine the tolerability, effectiveness, and safety of apixaban in prevention of thrombolic events in patients with advanced or metastatic cancer on prescribed chemotherapy for more than 90 days [63]. In this randomized double-blind study 12-week administration of apixaban (5, 10, or 20 mg once daily, n=95 overall) was compared to placebo (n=30). The primary outcome was either major bleeding or clinically relevant non-major bleeding and secondary outcomes included VTE and grade III or higher adverse events related to the study drug. Although the study appeared to show a favorable safety profile for apixaban, it was underpowered to draw any reliable conclusions and further phase III evaluation of apixaban in this setting would be appropriate [63].

A further phase III randomized trial, ADOPT, compared the safety and efficacy of apixaban with enoxaparin in preventing DVT and PE in patients hospitalized with congestive heart failure, acute respiratory failure, infection (without septic shock), acute rheumatic disorder, or inflammatory bowel disease [59]. A total of 6528 subjects underwent randomization, 4495 of whom could be evaluated for the primary efficacy outcome: 2211 in the apixaban group and 2284 in the enoxaparin group. The primary outcome was the composite of VTE or VTE-related death, whereas secondary outcome measures included all-cause mortality, major hemorrhage, and clinically relevant nonmajor hemorrhage. Among the patients who could be evaluated, 2.71% in the apixaban group and 3.06% in the enoxaparin group met the criteria for the primary efficacy outcome (relative risk with apixaban, 0.87; 95% CI, 0.62–1.23; P=0.44). Major bleeding occurred in 0.47% of the patients in the apixaban group and in 0.19% of the patients in the enoxaparin group. The investigators therefore concluded that in medically ill patients, an extended course of thromboprophylaxis with apixaban was not superior to a shorter course with enoxaparin and was associated with significantly more major bleeding events than was enoxaparin [59].

Treatment of venous thrombosis

Investigation of the utility of apixaban for the treatment of patients with VTE started with the phase II Botticelli DVT dose-ranging clinical trial [63]. In this study 520 patients with symptomatic DVT were randomized to receive apixaban (5 mg or 10 mg twice daily or 20 mg four-times daily) or traditional treatment with LMWH or fondaparinux followed by VKA. After management for 84–91 days, no significant difference was reported between the treatments in the rate of occurrence of the primary outcome, a composite of symptomatic recurrent VTE and asymptomatic deterioration of bilateral compression ultrasound or perfusion lung scan (4.7% for apixaban and 4.2% in control patients) [64]. The primary outcome rates for the tested apixaban doses were 6.0% for 5.0 mg twice daily, 5.6% for 10.0 mg twice daily, and 2.6% for 20.0 mg once daily. The principal safety outcome (a composite of major and clinically relevant nonmajor hemorrhage) developed at a similar rate in the apixaban-treated patients (7.3%) and the control group (7.9%). The principal safety outcome rates for the tested apixaban doses were 8.6% for 5.0 mg twice daily, 4.5% for 10.0 mg twice daily, and 7.3% for 20 mg once daily.

In the Phase III multicenter, randomized AMPLIFY study (NCT00643201) apixaban is being compared with the conventional treatment (enoxaparin/warfarin) in 3625 patients with DVT. Apixaban starting at 10 mg twice daily for 7 days is followed by a 5 mg twice-daily dose for 6 months. The primary outcome measures are the recurrence of VTE events or death; secondary outcome measures include the incidence of hemorrhage. Additionally, the AMPLIFY-EXT trial assessed the efficacy and safety of apixaban in preventing VTE recurrence or death in 2438 patients with clinical diagnosis of DVT or PE who have already completed their standard treatment for DVT or PE [65]. Patients received apixaban (2.5 or 5.0 mg twice daily) or placebo for 12 months. The study found that VTE or death from venous thromboembolism occurred in 8.8% of patients who received placebo, as compared with 1.7% who were received 2.5 mg of apixaban (95% CI 5.0-9.3) and 1.7% who were receiving 5 mg of apixaban (95% CI 4.9-9.1; $P<0.001$ for both) [65].

Acute coronary syndrome

The phase II APPRAISE-1 clinical trial evaluated the safety of apixaban in 1715 patients with recent ACS. Patients were randomized to receive apixaban (2.5 mg twice daily or 10.0 mg once daily) or placebo for 26 weeks. The primary outcome was the incidence of major or clinically relevant nonmajor hemorrhage; the secondary outcome was a composite of cardiovascular death, nonfatal myocardial infarction, severe recurrent ischemia, or ischemic stroke. The investigators reported a dose-related increase in bleeding compared with placebo (apixaban 2.5 mg twice daily: HR, 1.78; 95% CI 0.91-3.48; $P=0.09$; 10 mg once daily: HR, 2.45; 95% CI, 1.31–4.61; $P=0.005$) and a trend toward a reduction in ischemic events with the addition of apixaban to antiplatelet therapy in patients with recent ACS [60]. Whether apixaban can improve outcome in patients after an ACS was further investigated in the phase III trial APPRAISE-2. This trial was a randomized, double-blind, placebo-controlled clinical trial comparing apixaban, at a dose of 5 mg twice daily, with placebo, in addition to standard antiplatelet therapy, in patients with a recent ACS and at least two additional risk factors for recurrent ischemic events. The trial was terminated prematurely due to an increase in major bleeding events with apixaban in the absence of a counterbalancing reduction in recurrent ischemic events [61].

Emerging factor Xa inhibitors

The range of oral factor Xa inhibitors that have reached advanced stages of clinical development is increasing, reflecting interest in the high clinical potential of this pharmaceutical group.

Edoxaban

Edoxaban selectively inhibits factor Xa with high affinity (K_i 0.56 nmol/L). In rat models edoxaban was able to inhibit both arterial and venous thrombosis in the same dose range; in contrast, fondaparinux requires 100-fold higher concentrations to inhibit arterial rather than venous thrombosis

[66]. Data from animal models suggest that edoxaban may have a wider therapeutic range than UFH, LMWH, and warfarin, with a lower propensity for hemorrhage [67]. Edoxaban was also shown to potentiate the effects of the ticlopidine and tissue plasminogen activator in rat thrombosis models, suggesting that a combination therapy comprising edoxaban and either of these agents may be clinically useful [68]. In a phase I study in healthy males, a single 60 mg dose of edoxaban inhibited factor Xa activity, prolonged both the prothrombin time and activated partial thromboplastin time, and reduced in vitro venous and arterial thrombus formation [69]. The antifactor Xa activity of edoxaban peaks 1.5 hours after administration and lasts for up to 12 hours, with antithrombotic effects persisting for approximately 5 hours, suggesting that it has potential for once-daily dosing. There are two completed phase II dose-finding studies of edoxaban for the prevention of VTE after THR, NCT00107900 [25] and NCT00398216. In the study by Raskob et al, 903 patients were randomized to oral edoxaban (15, 30, 60, or 90 mg once daily) or subcutaneous dalteparin once daily (initial dose 2,500 IU, subsequent doses 5,000 IU) [25]. Both medications were started 6–8 hours after surgery and administered for 7–10 days. Data from 776 participants were included into the primary efficacy analysis. The primary efficacy endpoint of total VTE was significantly lower in subjects treated with edoxaban (28.2%, 21.2%, 15.2%, and 10.6% for 15, 30, 60, and 90 mg doses of edoxaban, respectively) than in those receiving dalteparin (43.8%, $P<0.005$). No significant difference between the drugs was seen in the primary safety outcome of major and clinically relevant non-major bleeding. Edoxaban was approved in Japan in April 2011 for the prevention of VTE following lower-limb orthopedic surgery. This approval was supported by data from two pivotal, randomized, double-blind, multicenter, phase III trials in knee surgery (NCT01181102) and hip surgery (NCT01181167). These trials compared edoxaban 30 mg once-daily with enoxaparin. In both trials, edoxaban was non-inferior to enoxaparin in the prevention of asymptomatic and symptomatic DVT and symptomatic PE.

A global phase III study, the HOKUSAI VTE trial (NCT00986154), investigating the safety and efficacy of edoxaban in the treatment and prevention of recurrent VTE in patients with DVT and/or PE is ongoing.

The edoxaban program for stroke prevention in AF has now been extended to a phase III trial, with 16,500 patients to be recruited in the ENGAGE AF-TIMI 48 study [70].

LY517717

LY517717 is a factor Xa inhibitor with an inhibitory rate constant (K_i) for factor Xa of 4.6–6.6 nmol/L and an oral bioavailability of 25–82%. It is eliminated mainly by the fecal route, with an elimination half-life of approximately 25 hours in healthy subjects [26]. In a phase II, randomized, double-blind, dose escalation study a dosing range of LY517717 25–150 mg once daily versus enoxaparin 40 mg once daily was tested in 511 patients undergoing TKR or THR [26]. The primary efficacy endpoint was the incidence of VTE at the end of treatment (6–10 days), and safety endpoints were the incidences of major and minor hemorrhage at 30 days after treatment initiation. Three lower doses of LY517717 were stopped due to lack of efficacy, and the three higher doses (100, 125, and 150 mg) were noninferior to enoxaparin (17.1–24.0% versus 22.2% with enoxaparin for the efficacy endpoint). The three higher LY517717 doses were associated with lower incidences of major hemorrhage (0.0–0.9% versus 1.1% with enoxaparin) and minor hemorrhage (0.0–1.0% versus 2.2% with enoxaparin). Gender and creatinine clearance were found to affect LY517717 exposure and may be partly responsible for the reported intra-individual variability of 35%. Information about any further clinical development of LY517717 is currently unavailable.

Betrixaban

Betrixaban (PRT-054021) specifically and reversibly inhibits factor Xa with a K_i of 0.117 nmol/L. It has a bioavailability of 47% and a half-life of 19 hours, and is excreted almost unchanged in bile. Betrixaban has demonstrated antithrombotic activity in animal models and in human blood and is well tolerated in healthy individuals across a wide range of doses. Betrixaban has been investigated in phase II trials for VTE prevention in patients after major joint surgery (EXPERT) [23] and for stroke prevention in patients with AF (EXPLORE-Xa) [24].

References

1   Mackman N. Triggers, targets and treatments for thrombosis. *Nature*. 2008;451:914-918.

2   Di Nisio M, Middeldorp S, Büller HR. Direct thrombin inhibitors. *N Engl J Med*. 2005;353:1028-1040.

3   Wallentin L, Wilcox RG, Weaver WD, et al; ESTEEM Investigators. Oral ximelagatran for secondary prophylaxis after myocardial infarction: the ESTEEM randomised controlled trial. *Lancet*. 2003;362:789-797.

4   Fiessinger JN, Huisman MV, Davidson BL, et al; THRIVE Treatment Study Investigators. Ximelagatran vs low-molecular-weight heparin and warfarin for the treatment of deep vein thrombosis: a randomized trial. *JAMA*. 2005;293:681-689.

5   Agnelli G, Eriksson BI, Cohen AT, et al; on behalf of the EXTEND Study Group. Safety assessment of new antithrombotic agents: Lessons from the EXTEND study on ximelagatran. *Thromb Res*. 2009;123:488-497.

6   Wienen W, Stassen JM, Priepke H, et al. Effects of the direct thrombin inhibitor dabigatran and its orally active prodrug, dabigatran etexilate, on thrombus formation and bleeding time in rats. *Thromb Haemost*. 2007;98:333-338.

7   Stangier J, Stahle H, Rathgen K, Fuhr R. Pharmacokinetics and pharmacodynamics of the direct oral thrombin inhibitor dabigatran in healthy elderly subjects. *Clin Pharmacokinet*. 2008;47:47-59.

8   Stangier J, Rathgen K, Stahle H, et al. The pharmacokinetics, pharmacodynamics and tolerability of dabigatran etexilate, a new oral direct thrombin inhibitor, in healthy male subjects. *Br J Clin Pharmacol*. 2007;64:292-303.

9   Gross PL, Weitz JI. New anticoagulants for treatment of venous thromboembolism. *Arterioscler Thromb Vasc Biol*. 2008;28:380-386.

10 Eriksson BI, Dahl OE, Ahnfelt L, et al. Dose escalating safety study of a new oral direct thrombin inhibitor, dabigatran etexilate, in patients undergoing total hip replacement: BISTRO I. *J Thromb Haemost*. 2004;2:1573-1580.

11 Eriksson BI, Dahl OE, Büller HR, et al; BISTRO II Study Group. A new oral direct thrombin inhibitor, dabigatran etexilate, compared with enoxaparin for prevention of thromboembolic events following total hip or knee replacement: the BISTRO II randomized trial. *J Thromb Haemost*. 2005;3:103-111.

12 Eriksson BI, Dahl OE, Rosencher N, et al; RE-MODEL Study Group. Oral dabigatran etexilate vs. subcutaneous enoxaparin for the prevention of venous thromboembolism after total knee replacement: the RE-MODEL randomized trial. *J Thromb Haemost*. 2007;5:2178-2185.

13 Eriksson BI, Dahl OE, Huo MH, et al; RE-NOVATE II Study Group. Oral dabigatran versus enoxaparin for thromboprophylaxis after primary total hip arthroplasty (RE-NOVATE II*). A randomised, double-blind, non-inferiority trial. *Thromb Haemost*. 2011;105:721-729.

14 RE-MOBILIZE Writing Committee, Ginsberg JS, Davidson BL, Comp PC, et al. Oral thrombin inhibitor dabigatran etexilate vs North American enoxaparin regimen for prevention of venous thromboembolism after knee arthroplasty surgery. *J Arthroplasty*.2009;24:1-9.

15 Eriksson BI, Dahl OE, Rosencher N, et al; RE-NOVATE Study Group. Dabigatran etexilate versus enoxaparin for prevention of venous thromboembolism after total hip replacement: a randomised, double-blind, non-inferiority trial. *Lancet*. 2007;370:949-956.

16 Colwell CW, Spiro TE. Efficacy and safety of enoxaparin to prevent deep vein thrombosis after hip arthroplasty. *Clin Orthop Relat Res*. 1995;319:215.

17 Schulman S, Kearon C, Kakkar AK, et al; RE-COVER Study Group. Dabigatran versus warfarin in the treatment of acute venous thromboembolism. *N Engl J Med*. 2009;361:2342-2352.

18 Ezekowitz MD, Reilly PA, Nehmiz G, et al. Dabigatran with or without concomitant aspirin compared with warfarin alone in patients with nonvalvular atrial fibrillation (PETRO Study). *Am J Cardiol*. 2007;100:1419-1426.

19 Connolly SJ, Ezekowitz MD, Yusuf S, et al. RE-LY Steering Committee and Investigators. Dabigatran versus warfarin in patients with atrial fibrillation. *N Engl J Med*. 2009;361:1139-1131.

20 Oldgren J, Budaj A, Granger CB, et al; RE-DEEM Investigators. Dabigatran vs. placebo in patients with acute coronary syndromes on dual antiplatelet therapy: a randomized, double-blind, phase II trial. *Eur Heart J.* 2011;32:2781-2789.

21 Schulman S, Baanstra D, Eriksson H, et al. Dabigatran versus placebo for extended maintenance therapy of venous thromboembolism. ISTH 2011; July 25, 2011; Kyoto, Japan. Abstract O-MO-037.

22 Schulman S, Eriksson H, Goldhaber SZ, et al. Dabigatran or warfarin for extended maintenance therapy of venous thromboembolism. ISTH 2011; July 28, 2011; Kyoto, Japan. Abstract O-TH-033.

23 Turpie AG, Bauer KA, Davidson BL, et al; EXPERT Study Group. A randomized evaluation of betrixaban, an oral factor Xa inhibitor, for prevention of thromboembolic events after total knee replacement (EXPERT). *Thromb Haemost.* 2009;101:68-76.

24 Connolly SJ, Ezekowitz MD, Diaz R, Hohnloser SH, Dorian P. A phase 2, randomized, parallel group, dose-finding, multicenter, multinational study of the safety, tolerability and pilot efficacy of three blinded doses of the oral factor Xa inhibitor betrixaban compared with open-label dose-adjusted warfarin in patients with non-valvular atrial fibrillation (EXPLORE-Xa). Presentation at the American College of Cardiology (ACC) 59th Annual Scientific Session; Atlanta, GA; 2010.

25 Raskob G, Cohen AT, Eriksson BI, et al. Oral direct factor Xa inhibition with edoxaban for thromboprophylaxis after elective total hip replacement. A randomised double-blind dose-response study. *Thromb Haemost.* 2010;104:642-649.

26 Agnelli G, Haas S, Ginsberg JS, et al. A phase II study of the oral factor Xa inhibitor LY517717 for the prevention of venous thromboembolism after hip or knee replacement. *J Thromb Haemost.* 2007;5:746-753.

27 Sabatine MS, Antman EM, Widimsky P, et al. Otamixaban for the treatment of patients with non-ST-elevation acute coronary syndromes (SEPIA-ACS1 TIMI 42): a randomised, double-blind, active-controlled, phase 2 trial. *Lancet.* 2009;374:787-795.

28 Kakar P, Watson T, Lip GYH. Drug evaluation: Rivaroxaban, an oral, direct inhibitor of activated Factor X. *Curr Opin Investig Drugs.* 2007;8:256-265.

29 Kubitza D, Becka M, Wensing G, et al. Safety, pharmacodynamics, and pharmacokinetics of BAY 59-7939 – an oral, direct Factor Xa inhibitor – after multiple dosing in healthy male subjects. *Eur J Clin Pharmacol.* 2005;61:873-880.

30 Gruber A, Marzec UM, Buetehorn U, Hanson S, Perzborn E. Potential of activated prothrombin complex concentrate and activated Factor VII to reverse the anticoagulant effects of rivaroxaban in primates. *Blood (ASH Annual Meeting Abstracts).* 2008;112:1307:abstract 3825.

31 Perzborn E, Trabandt A, Selbach K, Tinel H. Prothrombin complex concentrate reverses the effects of high-dose rivaroxaban in rats. *J Thromb Haemost.* 2009;7:379:abstract PP-MO-183.

32 Perzborn E, Roehrig S, Straub A, Kubitza D, Misselwitz F. The discovery and development of rivaroxaban, an oral, direct factor Xa inhibitor. *Nat Rev Drug Discov.* 2011;10:61-75.

33 Eriksson BI, Borris LC, Dahl OE, et al; ODIXa-HIP Study Investigators. A once-daily, oral, direct Factor Xa inhibitor, rivaroxaban (BAY 59-7939), for thromboprophylaxis after total hip replacement. *Circulation.* 2006;114:2374-2381.

34 Eriksson BI, Borris L, Dahl OE, et al; ODIXa-HIP Study Investigators. Oral, direct Factor Xa inhibition with BAY 59-7939 for the prevention of venous thromboembolism after total hip replacement. *J Thromb Haemost.* 2006;4:121-128.

35 Eriksson BI, Borris LC, Dahl OE, et al. Dose-escalation study of rivaroxaban (BAY 59-7939) – an oral, direct Factor Xa inhibitor – for the prevention of venous thromboembolism in patients undergoing total hip replacement. *Thromb Res.* 2007;120:685-693.

36 Turpie AG, Fisher WD, Bauer KA, et al; OdiXa-Knee Study Group. BAY 59-7939: an oral, direct factor Xa inhibitor for the prevention of venous thromboembolism in patients after total knee replacement. A phase II dose-ranging study. *J Thromb Haemost.* 2005;3:2479-2486.

37 Fisher WD, Eriksson BI, Bauer KA, et al. Rivaroxaban for thromboprophylaxis after orthopaedic surgery: pooled analysis of two studies. *Thromb Haemost.* 2007;97:931-937.

38 Eriksson BI, Borris LC, Friedman RJ, et al; RECORD1 Study Group. Rivaroxaban versus enoxaparin for thromboprophylaxis after hip arthroplasty. *N Engl J Med.* 2008;358:2765-2775.

39 Lassen MR, Ageno W, Borris LC, et al; RECORD3 Investigators. Rivaroxaban versus enoxaparin for thromboprophylaxis after total knee arthroplasty. *N Engl J Med.* 2008;358:2776-2786.

40 Kakkar AK, Brenner B, Dahl OE, et al; RECORD2 Investigators. Extended duration rivaroxaban versus short-term enoxaparin for the prevention of venous thromboembolism after total hip arthroplasty: a double-blind, randomised controlled trial. *Lancet.* 2008;372:31-39.

41 Turpie AG, Lassen MR, Davidson BL, et al; RECORD4 Investigators. Rivaroxaban versus enoxaparin for thromboprophylaxis after total knee arthroplasty (RECORD4): a randomised trial. *Lancet.* 2009;9676:1673-1680.

42 Cohen AT, Spiro TE, Büller HR, et al. Extended-duration rivaroxaban thromboprophylaxis in acutely ill medical patients: MAGELLAN study protocol. *J Thromb Thrombolysis.* 2011;31:407-416.

43 Agnelli G, Gallus A, Goldhaber SZ, et al; ODIXa-DVT Study Investigators. Treatment of proximal deep-vein thrombosis with the oral direct Factor Xa inhibitor rivaroxaban (BAY 59-7939): the ODIXa- DVT (oral direct Factor Xa inhibitor BAY 59-7939 in patients with acute symptomatic deep-vein thrombosis) study. *Circulation.* 2007;116:180-187.

44 Buller HR, Lensing AW, Prins MH, et al; EINSTEIN-DVT Dose-Ranging Study investigators. A dose-ranging study evaluating once-daily oral administration of the factor Xa inhibitor rivaroxaban in the treatment of patients with acute symptomatic deep vein thrombosis. The EINSTEIN- DVT Dose-Ranging Study. *Blood.* 2008;112:2242-2247.

45 The EINSTEIN-PE Investigators. Oral rivaroxaban for the treatment of symptomatic pulmonary embolism. *N Engl J Med.* 2012;366:1287-1297.

46 Romualdi E, Donadini MP, Ageno W. Oral rivaroxaban after symptomatic venous thromboembolism: the continued treatment study (EINSTEIN-extension study). *Expert Rev Cardiovasc Ther.* 2011;9:841-844.

47 EINSTEIN Investigators; Bauersachs R, Berkowitz SD, Brenner B, et al. Oral rivaroxaban for symptomatic venous thromboembolism. *N Engl J Med.* 2010;363:2499-2510.

48 Patel MR, Mahaffey KW, Garg J, et al; ROCKET AF Investigators. Rivaroxaban versus warfarin in nonvalvular atrial fibrillation. *N Engl J Med.* 2011;365:883-891.

49 Mega JL, Braunwald E, Wiviott SD, et al; ATLAS ACS 2–TIMI 51 Investigators. Rivaroxaban in patients with a recent acute coronary syndrome. *N Engl J Med.* 2012;366:9-19.

50 Hori M, Matsumoto M, Tanahashi N, et al. Rivaroxaban vs. warfarin in Japanese patients with atrial fibrillation. *Circ J.* 2012 Jun 5. [Epub ahead of print].

51 Wong PC, Crain EJ, Xin B, et al. Apixaban, an oral, direct and highly selective factor Xa inhibitor: in vitro, antithrombotic and antihemostatic studies. *J Thromb Haemost.* 2008;6:820-829.

52 Mega JL, Braunwald E, Mohanavelu S, et al; ATLAS ACS-TIMI 46 study group. Rivaroxaban versus placebo in patients with acute coronary syndromes (ATLAS ACS-TIMI 46): a randomised, double-blind, phase II trial. *Lancet.* 2009;374:29-38.

53 Shantsila E, Lip GY. Apixaban, an oral, direct inhibitor of activated Factor Xa. *Curr Opin Investig Drugs.* 2008;9:1020-1033.

54 Lassen MR, Raskob GE, Gallus A, Pineo G, Chen D, Portman RJ. Apixaban or enoxaparin for thromboprophylaxis after knee replacement. *N Engl J Med.* 2009;36:594-604.

55 Lassen MR, Raskob GE, Gallus A, et al; ADVANCE-2 Investigators. Apixaban versus enoxaparin for thromboprophylaxis after knee replacement (ADVANCE 2): a randomised double-blind trial. *Lancet.* 2010;375:807-815.

56 Lassen MR, Gallus A, Raskob GE, et al; ADVANCE-3 Investigators. Apixaban versus enoxaparin for thromboprophylaxis after hip replacement. *N Engl J Med.* 2010;363:2487-2498.

57 Granger CB, Alexander JH, McMurray JJ, et al; ARISTOTLE Committees and Investigators. Apixaban versus warfarin in patients with atrial fibrillation. *N Engl J Med.* 2011;365:981-992.

58 Connolly SJ, Eikelboom J, Joyner C, et al; AVERROES Steering Committee and Investigators. Apixaban in patients with atrial fibrillation. *N Engl J Med.* 2011;364:806-817.

59 Goldhaber SZ, Leizorovicz A, Kakkar AK, et al; ADOPT Trial Investigators. Apixaban versus enoxaparin for thromboprophylaxis in medically ill patients. *N Engl J Med.* 2011;365:2167-2177.

60 APPRAISE Steering Committee and Investigators; Alexander JH, Becker RC, Bhatt DL, et al. Apixaban, an oral, direct, selective factor Xa inhibitor, in combination with antiplatelet therapy after acute coronary syndrome: results of the Apixaban for Prevention of Acute Ischemic and Safety Events (APPRAISE) trial. *Circulation*. 2009;119:2877-2885.

61 APPRAISE-2 Investigators; Alexander JH, Lopes RD, James S, et al. Apixaban with antiplatelet therapy after acute coronary syndrome. *N Engl J Med*. 2011;365:699-708

62 Lassen MR, Davidson BL, Gallus A, Pineo G, Ansell J, Deitchman D. The efficacy and safety of apixaban, an oral, direct factor Xa inhibitor, as thromboprophylaxis in patients following total knee replacement. *J Thromb Haemost*. 2007;5:2368-2375.

63 Levine MN, Gu C, Liebman HA, et al. A randomized phase II trial of apixaban for the prevention of thromboembolism in patients with metastatic cancer. *J Thromb Haemost*. 2012;10:807-814.

64 Botticelli Investigators, Writing Committee; Buller H, Deitchman D, Prins M, et al. Efficacy and safety of the oral direct factor Xa inhibitor apixaban for symptomatic deep vein thrombosis. The Botticelli DVT dose-ranging study. *J Thromb Haemost*. 2008;6:1313-1318.

65 AMPLIFY-EXT Investigators; Agnelli G, Buller HR, Cohen A, et al. Apixaban for extended treatment of venous thromboembolism. N Engl J Med. 2013;368:699-708.Fukuda T, Matsumoto C, Honda Y, Sugiyama N, Morishima Y, Shibano T. Antithrombotic properties of DU-176b, a novel, potent and orally active direct Factor Xa inhibitor in rat models of arterial and venous thrombosis: comparison with fondaparinux, an antithrombin dependent Factor Xa inhibitor. *ASH Annual Meeting Abstracts*. 2004;104:1852.

66 Fukuda T, Matsumoto C, Honda Y, Sugiyama N, Morishima Y, Shibano T. Antithrombotic properties of DU-176b, a novel, potent and orally active direct Factor Xa inhibitor in rat models of arterial and venous thrombosis: comparison with fondaparinux, an antithrombin dependent Factor Xa inhibitor. *ASH Annual Meeting Abstracts*. 2004;104:1852.

67 Furugohri T, Honda Y, Matsumoto C, Isobe K, Sugiyama N, Morishima Y, Shibano T. Antithrombotic and hemorrhagic effects of DU-176b, a novel, potent and orally active direct Factor Xa inhibitor: a wider safety margin compared to heparins and warfarin. *ASH Annual Meeting Abstracts*. 2004;104:1851.

68 Morishima Y, Furugohri T, Honda Y, et al. Antithrombotic properties of DU-176b, a novel orally active Factor Xa inhibitor: inhibition of both arterial and venous thrombosis, and combination effects with other antithrombotic agents. *J Thromb Haemost*. 2005;3:abstract PO511.

69 Zafar MU, Gaztanga J, Velez M, et al. A phase-I study to assess the antithrombotic properties of DU-176b: an orally active direct Factor-Xa inhibitor. *J Am Coll Cardiol*. 2006;47:288A.

70 Daiichi Sankyo Inc. Global study to assess the safety and effectiveness of DU-176b vs standard practice of dosing with warfarin in patients with atrial fibrillation (EngageAFTIMI48) [ClinicalTrials.gov identifier NCT00781391]. US National Institutes of Health, ClinicalTrials.gov. Available at: www.clinicaltrials.gov. [Accessed June 13, 2013].

Chapter 6

Future directions

Eduard Shantsila, Gregory YH Lip

The large number of novel oral anticoagulants under clinical development reflects the huge clinical demand for such medicines and the desire of the pharmaceutical industry to respond to the as yet unmet needs of patients. Chronic life-long prevention of thromboembolic stroke in atrial fibrillation, an increasingly common cardiac arrhythmia, represents the largest need for oral anticoagulants, and they are required by millions of patients worldwide. Improvements in the diagnosis of venous thromboembolic events, such as pulmonary embolization, along with growing appreciation of their high prevalence and life-threatening nature, have increased the demand for convenient and reliable long-term anticoagulation.

In addition to having an irreplaceable role in venous thrombosis, the effectiveness of inhibitors of the coagulation cascade in clinical settings of arterial thrombosis, such as myocardial infarction and acute coronary syndromes, is being extensively evaluated. At present, antiplatelet drugs dominate in this field; however, it appears that continuous enhancement of the potency of antiplatelet agents has its own natural limits. Breaching of these limits may provide a certain amount of benefit in terms of prevention of thrombosis but it has a downside, as evidenced by the high rate of severe hemorrhage and even by the impairment of immune responses and activation of silent cancers. The process of arterial thrombosis, although initiated by the formation of predominantly platelet clots, has numerous links with coagulation factors and often includes a significant fibrin

G. Y. H. Lip and E. Shantsila (eds.), *Handbook of Oral Anticoagulation*, DOI: 10.1007/978-1-908517-96-8_6, © Springer Healthcare 2013

component. Consequently, parenteral anticoagulants, such as heparin, have become an important part of management of patients with arterial thrombosis. Not surprisingly, several novel oral anticoagulants are being tested on patients with acute coronary syndromes.

The promise of convenient long-term anticoagulation may itself lengthen the list of potential indications for novel anticoagulants. For example, patients with various chronic conditions, such as heart failure, certain cancers, and prolonged immobilization, are known to bear high risks of thrombotic complications and thus may benefit from anticoagulant therapy if it can be provided conveniently and safely.

What would be the characteristics of the ideal anticoagulant? To make it convenient for long-term use, it would be available for oral administration. The onset of full anticoagulant action would be quick and stable throughout the day (ideally with a once-daily regimen). The anticoagulant effects would be predictable with fixed doses and would not require routine laboratory monitoring. The drug would have, if any, minimal interactions with other medicines and food. And ultimately, it must have a good safety profile in terms of risks of hemorrhage and possible effects on other organs (eg, the kidney or liver).

Can such a drug be developed in the near future? Most probably, the answer will be yes. Three novel oral anticoagulants, the direct thrombin inhibitor dabigatran etexilate and the factor Xa inhibitors rivaroxaban and apixaban, have already successfully completed phase III trials for indications requiring long-term anticoagulation. These drugs largely correspond to the requirements of an ideal anticoagulant. Furthermore, as they all participate in late stages of the coagulation cascade, their inhibition allows disruption of both the intrinsic and the extrinsic pathways; their high antithrombotic efficacy stems from this 'double' action. The results of further large clinical trials of these agents in a wider range of indications are eagerly awaited.